An Atlas of
URO-ONCOLOGY

THE ENCYCLOPEDIA OF VISUAL MEDICINE SERIES

An Atlas of
URO-ONCOLOGY

Roger S. Kirby

Professor of Urology

St. George's Hospital

London, UK

Foreword by

Jerome P. Richie, MD

Elliott C. Cutler Professor of Surgery

Harvard Medical School

Chairman, Harvard Program in Urology

The Parthenon Publishing Group

International Publishers in Medicine, Science & Technology

A CRC PRESS COMPANY

BOCA RATON   LONDON   NEW YORK   WASHINGTON, D.C.

Published in the USA by
The Parthenon Publishing Group Inc.
345 Park Avenue South, 10th Floor
New York
NY 10010
USA

Published in the UK by
The Parthenon Publishing Group
23–25 Blades Court
Deodar Road
London SW15 2NU
UK

Library of Congress Cataloging-in-Publication Data
Data available on request

British Library Cataloguing in Publication Data
Data available on request

ISBN 1-85070-614-X

First published in 2002

Composition by The Parthenon Publishing Group
Illustrated by Dee McLean, London, UK
Color reproduction by Graphic Reproductions, UK
Printed and bound by T. G. Hostench S.A., Spain

Contents

List of illustrations

RENAL CANCER

BLADDER CANCER

TESTICULAR CANCER

PENILE CANCER

Foreword

The increasing complexity of urological oncology necessitates ever-increasing diligence in order to understand the rapid evolutionary and revolutionary changes that are occurring. The concept of diagrams and algorithms allows the reader the luxury to develop a snapshot to quickly grasp the big picture.

This Atlas has succeeded admirably in capturing the essence of complex procedures. Cutting-edge technology is included, with timely topics such as molecular biology – including cell adhesion molecules, the caspase apoptosis pathway, and angiogenesis, as well as signal transduction.

Each of the five urological cancers – prostate, bladder, renal, testis, and penis – is detailed, including treatment options, surgical technique, and management of advanced disease, along with excellent bibliographies.

This atlas can serve as an important reference tool for urological oncologists, radiation oncologists, medical oncologists, and residents and fellows in training. The carefully designed bibliography serves as an updated reference list for further in-depth study.

Jerome P. Richie, MD
Elliott C. Cutler Professor of Surgery
Harvard Medical School
Chairman, Harvard Program in Urology

Preface

We are all, it has aptly been said, drowning in a sea of information, but thirsting for knowledge. Who (apart from those sitting examinations) in this busy 'information age' has time to plough through a two- or three-volume textbook of uro-oncology? In this Atlas, therefore, I have tried to distil the essence of what is potentially a vast subject. Since pictures speak louder than words (and convey very much more information), I have tried to keep the text to a minimum and focus exclusively on the most commonly encountered tumors of the prostate, kidney, bladder, testis and penis.

Decisions can be difficult. Almost every day, the uro-oncologist, in informed discussion with his or her patient, has to decide which of a selection of investigations and treatment strategies to employ. In this book, state-of the-art decision diagrams for all the common uro-oncological diseases are provided to facilitate this process.

A book like this doesn't just happen, it has to be made to happen. Consequently, I would like to thank Dee McLean, who worked so hard to produce the illustrations, Nicola Bentham, who helped to prepare the manuscript, and Jean Wright and her outstanding production team at Parthenon. Many of the histopathology illustrations were kindly provided by The Institute of Urology, University College London. Dr David Rickards generously supplied many of the radiological images, for which I am most grateful.

Roger Kirby

1

Molecular basis of urological cancers

Although the precise pathways that eventually result in cancer of the kidney, bladder, prostate and testis are still to be defined, the recent revolution in molecular genetics is providing us with an ever-clearer insight into their underlying subcellular basis. Induction and progression of urological cancers can generally be considered an evolutionary process. Each cancer develops as an independent sequence of events, in which mutations are selected because they provide an advantage to the outgrowth of the tumor, usually by increasing its rate of cell division. The process is stepwise, and each mutation must occur within the clone that is the expansion of the previous mutation. The term 'mutation' includes any stable change in gene expression, namely epigenetic events. These are now recognized as frequently consisting of changes in methylation which affect gene expression, and which are effectively as stable

as the less common 'true' mutations, namely alterations in the sequence of purines and pyrimidines that make up the deoxyribonucleic acid (DNA).

The specific causes of either DNA methylation or changes in nucleotide sequence in a given urological tumor type are as yet still to be discovered. A genetic predisposition to prostate cancer has been proposed to be the result of the deletion of a tumor suppressor gene in the region of chromosome 1q23–24 (Figure 1). Another candidate gene is located on the X chromosome. Other prostate cancer susceptibility genes seem certain to be discovered in the ongoing genome-wide search.

Although around 9% of prostate cancers may result from some inherited predisposition, the remaining 90% or so are probably the result of random mutations acquired throughout life. The same is probably true of other urological malignancies.

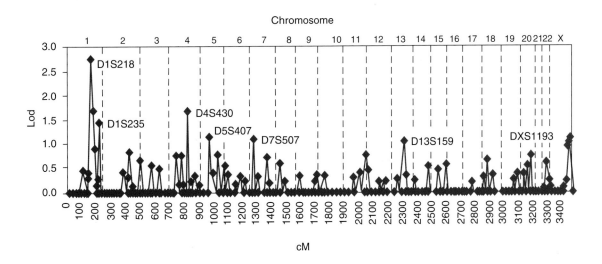

Figure 1 The HPC1 gene is demonstrated on lod analysis to reside on chromosome 1q

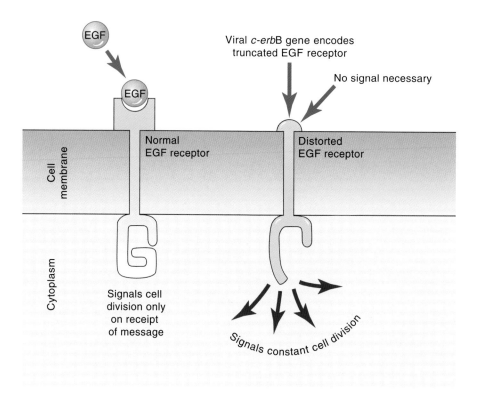

Figure 2 The *cErbB* oncogene in its normal and mutated variants

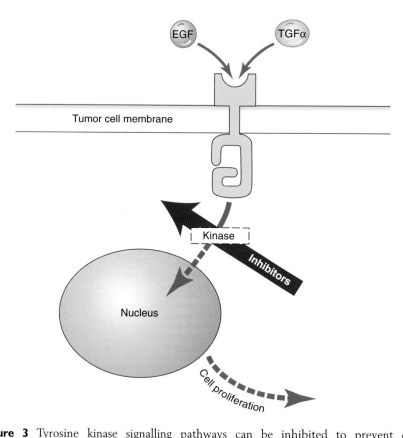

Figure 3 Tyrosine kinase signalling pathways can be inhibited to prevent cancer progresssion

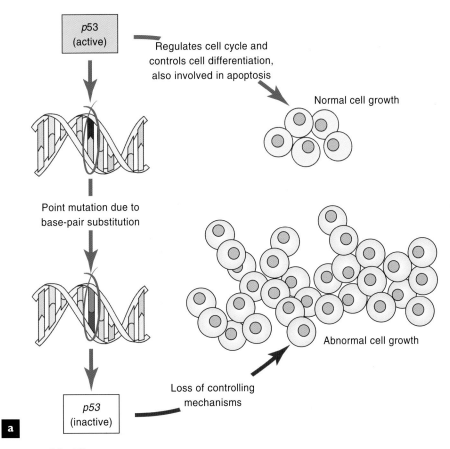

Figure 4 (a) *p53* tumor suppressor gene

These include the activation of oncogenes, such as *c Erb-B* , the classic oncogene, which, when activated, encodes a mutated version of the epidermal growth factor (EGF) receptor. This truncated receptor has lost the extracellular component which normally binds to EGF (Figure 2). Thus, instead of responding appropriately to its signal molecule, the mutated receptor stimulates continuing cell division and uncontrolled growth through the tyrosine kinase signalling pathways (Figure 3).

Other important steps involve the deactivation of tumor suppressor genes. Currently, the best characterized examples are *p53* (Figure 4) and the retinoblastoma gene, but other genes are unquestionably involved. Oncogenes and tumor suppressor genes apart, carcinogenesis also involves loss of cell-to-cell adhesion which normally maintains tissue structure and discourages cell migration. Specifically, deletion of E-cadherin or β-catenin appears to promote cell motility and this predisposes towards metastasis (Figure 5).

Some years ago, it was proposed that one important defence against malignancy was the body's own

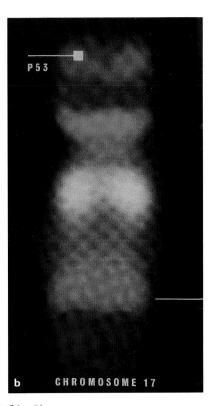

Figure 4 (b) *p53* tumor suppressor gene

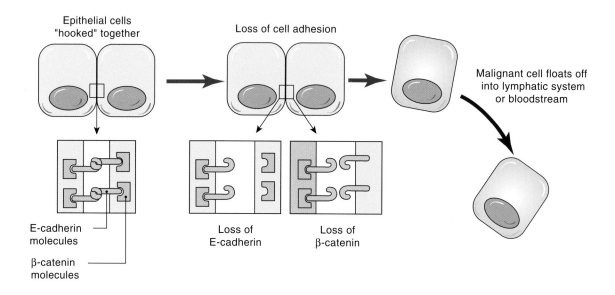

Figure 5 E-cadherin and β-catenin cell adherence molecules promote cell adhesion. When these proteins are lost, cells may detach and metastasis occurs

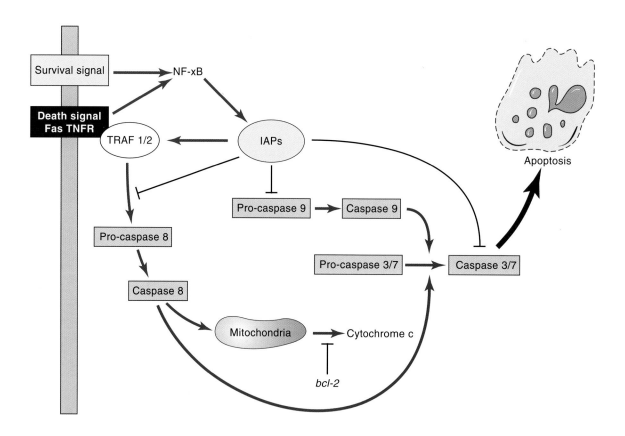

Figure 6 The caspase apoptosis pathways controlling programmed cell death. Inhibitors of apoptosis proteins (IAPs) and products of the *bcl-2* anti-apoptosis gene protect against the apoptotic signal of the *fas* gene and the effects of stimulation of tumor necrosis factor receptors (TNFR)

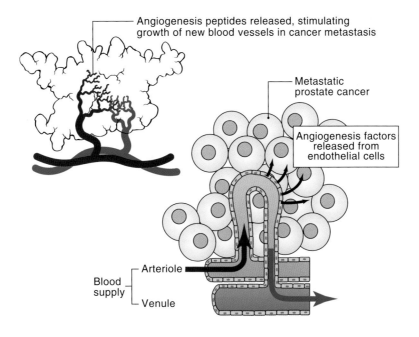

Figure 7 Angiogenesis and development of metastases

immunological surveillance. A more recent discovery is the apoptosis system of programmed cell death, which involves the proteolytic enzymes and the *bax* and *bcl-2* genes. Recent evidence suggests that many malignant cells undergo apoptosis with reabsorption of their constituent parts before they are capable of becoming a threat to the organism itself. The caspase pathways facilitating apoptosis have recently been characterized (Figure 6).

Once a cancer has formed in the kidney, bladder, prostate or testes, it usually develops first as a nodule (or nodules) and then develops the capacity to spread to local lymphatics or more distant sites, such as lungs or bone. In order for either the primary or secondary tumors to grow beyond 5 mm or so in size, the tumor has to induce its own blood supply – this process is known as angiogenesis (Figure 7). Evidence is accumulating that angiogenesis is a critical event in the genesis of both primary and metastatic urological malignancies.

The exciting feature of our ever-expanding detailed knowledge base of the molecular basis of urological cancer is its tremendous potential therapeutic value. Manipulation of oncogenes, tumor suppressor genes, cell adherence molecules and the molecular controls over angiogenesis may before too long become important components of our therapeutic armoury against many urological cancers.

FURTHER READING

DeWolf WC, Rukstalis DB. Principles of molecular genetics. In Walsh PC, Retik AB, Barracott-Vaughan E, Wein AJ, eds. *Campbells Urology*, 7th edn. Philadelphia: Saunders, 1998:3–48

McEleny KR, Watson RWG, Fitzpatrick JM. Defining a role for the inhibitors of apoptosis proteins in prostate cancer. *Prostate Cancer and Prostatic Diseases* 2001;4:28–32

Neal DE. Cancer, tumour suppressor genes and oncogenes. In Mundy AR, Fitzpatrick JM, Neal DE, George NJR, eds. *Scientific Basis of Urology*. Oxford: Isis Medical Media, 1999: 301–17

2

Prostate cancer

Prostate cancer is the most common urological malignancy and, in many ways, the most enigmatic. In Europe and the USA combined, it results in almost 100 000 deaths per year. After a steady rise in mortality during the 1980s and 1990s, recent years have witnessed a 7% reduction in prostate cancer deaths in the USA – an observation that some ascribe to the widespread implementation of prostate-specific antigen (PSA) screening and an active intervention program, although other factors, such as dietary modification and other lifestyle changes, may also be important.

RISK FACTORS FOR PROSTATE CANCER

Age is the single greatest risk factor for prostate cancer. No other malignancy shows such a steep positive correlation with age (Figure 8). Family history is a second factor, especially if one or more first-degree relatives are affected with an early age of onset (Figure 9). Consumption of saturated animal fat is an important modifiable risk factor (Figure 10). The explanation for this may be the oxidative damage to prostate cells from the free radicals produced during fat metabolism. A further component

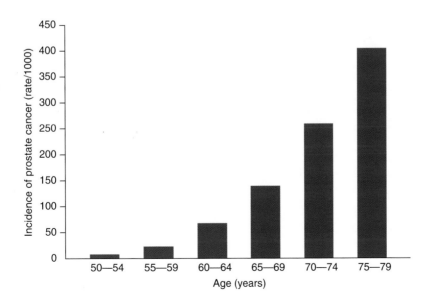

Figure 8 Age and prostate cancer incidence

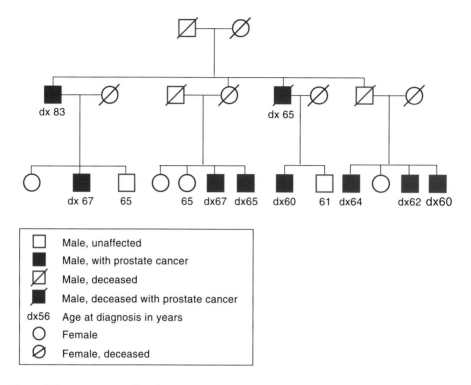

Figure 9 Prostate cancer family tree

is exposure to sunlight, which appears somehow protective – the prostate cancer risk rises in relation to distance from the equator. A protective influence of vitamin D has been postulated as the explanation. In addition, dietary supplements such as vitamin E and selenium, as well as intake of various specific vegetables, including tomatoes, which contain lycopenes, may reduce prostate cancer risk, perhaps by reducing oxidative stress on prostatic epithelial cells. Other, more effective chemopreventative agents will undoubtedly be discovered or developed.

DIAGNOSIS

Traditionally, prostate cancer has been diagnosed on the basis of symptoms which develop, either as a result of local infiltration of the gland or adjacent structures, causing voiding symptoms, or pain or other symptoms stemming from metastatic spread, most often to bones. Currently, however, as a result of increasingly widespread PSA testing, the disease is detected at a much earlier, often impalpable, asymptomatic stage. While this offers a much greater opportunity for cure, it also presents clinicians with

a therapeutic dilemma, since it is clear that not every prostate cancer detected will necessarily pose a threat to the life expectancy of the individual affected. Randomized studies of PSA screening are underway both in America and in Europe and should eventually confirm or refute the suggestion that early detection by PSA screening can indeed save lives.

Prostate-specific antigen is a glycoprotein secreted almost exclusively by the glandular epithelium of the prostate, the function of which is to liquefy semen after ejaculation (Figure 11). Normally, only a tiny proportion (less than one millionth) is absorbed into the bloodstream, where it is mainly bound, either to antichymotrypsin (ACT) or α-macroglobulin. Immunoassays can measure the quantities of both bound and unbound (so-called 'free') PSA in the serum. In prostate cancer, because of disruption to the basal cell layers and basement membrane, larger quantities of PSA enter the bloodstream (Figure 12) and the level of unbound PSA falls. As a consequence, serum PSA values and the ratio of free to total PSA provide valuable means of assessing the risk of a given man harboring adenocarcinoma within the gland.

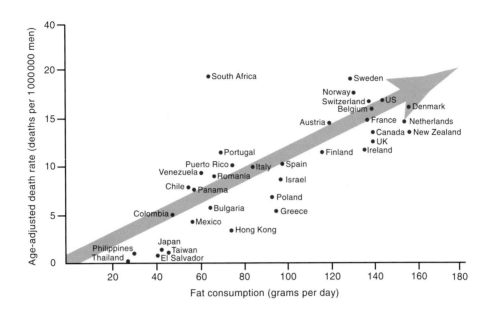

Figure 10 Fat consumption as a risk factor for prostate cancer by country

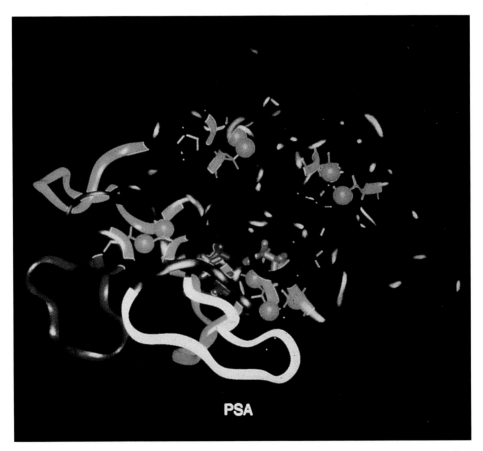

Figure 11 Molecular model of prostate-specific antigen (PSA)

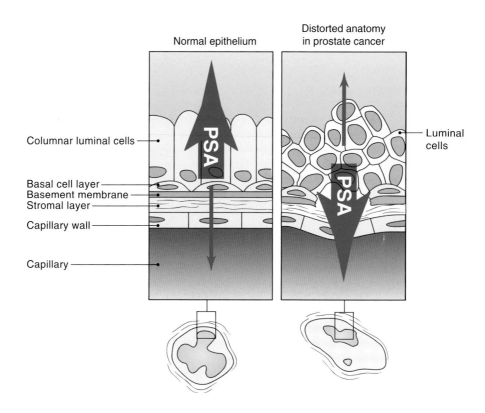

Figure 12 Production of prostate-specific antigen (PSA) by prostatic epithelium

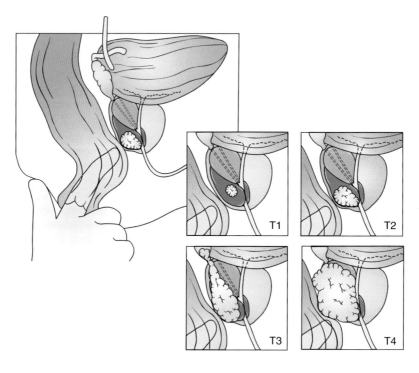

Figure 13 Clinical stage of prostate cancer as judged by digital rectal examination

In men with a raised PSA (usually taken as > 4 ng/ml) or other symptoms or signs of prostate cancer, a careful digital rectal examination (DRE) should be performed. Sometimes, a distinct nodule can be palpated; alternatively, one lobe or the entire gland may feel indurated. The clinical stage on DRE (Figure 13), taken in conjunction with the serum PSA value and the Gleason score, can provide an estimate of the probability of extraprostatic extension of the disease.

Assuming that the individual affected has a reasonable life expectancy (i.e. that a diagnosis of prostate cancer is likely to be of some clinical utility), a transrectal ultrasound (TRUS)-guided biopsy of the prostate is usually organized. This procedure is performed under antibiotic cover and with local anesthesia, and generally six, but sometimes as many as 12, systematic core biopsies of the gland are taken (Figure 14). In men with PSA values > 10 ng/ml, targetted biopsies of the seminal vesicles may also be obtained.

Histological assessment of prostatic tissue derived from TRUS-guided biopsy may confirm the presence of adenocarcinoma. A Gleason score can be calculated from the sum of the two most predominant tumor patterns, each of which is assigned a number from 1 to 5 according to the degree of glandular differentiation (1 = well differentiated with recognizable gland formation, 5 = poorly differentiated with amorphous sheets of cancer cells) (Figures 15–20). In addition, prostatic acini are assessed for the presence or absence of the premalignant change known as prostatic intraepithelial neoplasia (PIN). In this condition, estimated to be associated with concomitant cancer in 30–50% of cases, prostatic epithelial cells lose their normal columnar polarity (Figures 21 and 22). In spite of this, the basal layer remains intact and no invasion, which is the hallmark of true malignancy, is apparent. In cases of doubt, immunocytochemistry can be used to detect cytokeratins, seen in the basal but not the luminal cells (e.g. LP34, CK5 + 6), to highlight the basal layer (Figure 23). Special staining for PSA itself can also be helpful in confirming the prostatic origin of a secondary tumor in, for example, a lymph node (Figure 24).

In men whose TRUS-guided biopsies have revealed adenocarcinoma, a careful explanation of the findings and their implications is required. Depending on the PSA value, DRE and TRUS biopsy findings, further staging studies may be required.

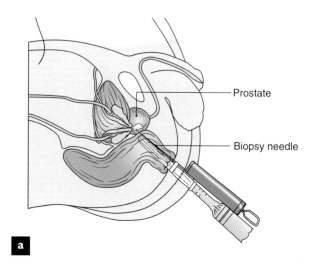

a

Prostate

Biopsy needle

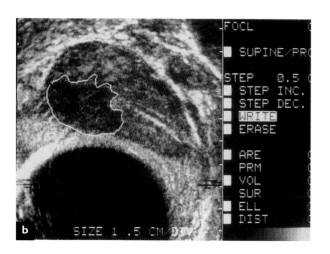

b   SIZE 1 .5 CM/DIV

FOCL
SUPINE/PR(
STEP   0.5
STEP INC.
STEP DEC.
WRITE
ERASE
ARE
PRM
VOL
SUR
ELL
DIST

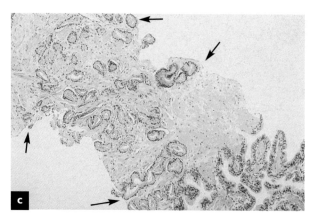

c

Figure 14 (a) TRUS-guided biopsy of the prostate;(b) ultrasound image; and (c) biopsy showing adenocarcinoma, Gleason 3 + 3 above left (arrow) and benign tissue lower right

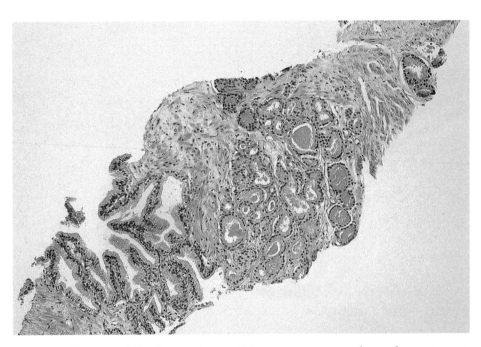

Figure 15 Gleason grade 2 adenocarcinoma of the prostate: compact focus of separate acini

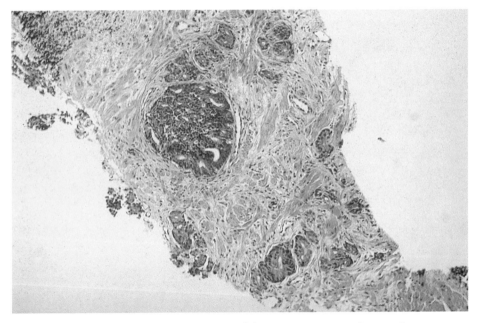

Figure 16 Gleason grade 3 adenocarcinoma of the prostate: scattered acini of varying size and a small circumscribed cribriform focus

These include magnetic resonance imaging (MRI) to evaluate local spread (Figures 25 and 26), as well as computerized tomography (CT), to estimate the risk of lymphatic involvement (Figure 27), and radionucleide bone scanning to detect the presence of bone metastases (Figure 28). In men with only mildly elevated PSA values (4–10 ng/ml), the probability of a positive result is low (Figure 29); conse-

quently, many urologists now omit some or all of these investigations and simply proceed to therapy of curative intent (see decision diagrams in Figure 30).

TREATMENT OPTIONS

Because of the lack of completed randomized, controlled trials, the treatment of prostate cancer,

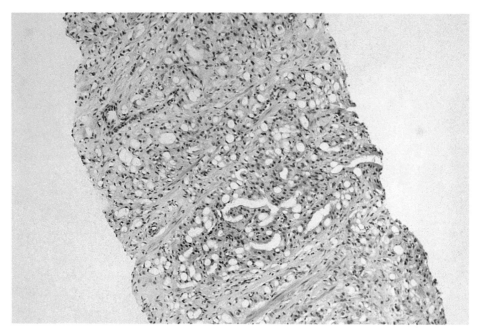

Figure 17 Gleason grade 4 adenocarcinoma of the prostate: fused acini producing a cribriform growth pattern

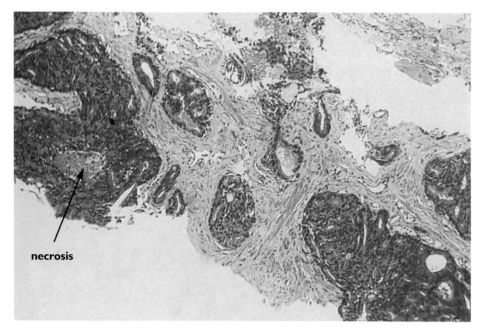

Figure 18 Gleason sum score 4 + 5 adenocarcinoma of the prostate: large, irregular cribriform islands of tumor with central necrosis

especially localized prostate cancer, remains controversial. In general, in the face of uncertainty, most clinicians engage the patient in a detailed discussion of the available treatment options, so that an informed decision, which takes account of individual patient preferences, can be reached. Treatment options vary according to whether the patient has localized disease, locally advanced disease or metastatic prostatic malignancy.

LOCALIZED PROSTATE CANCER

For men presenting with clinically localized prostate cancer, a number of treatment options exist.

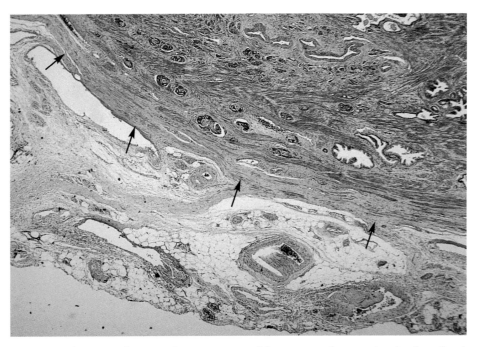

Figure 19 Gleason grade 3 + 4 adenocarcinoma of the prostate shown to be gland-confined in a radical prostatectomy specimen. The arrows indicate the edge of the prostate gland

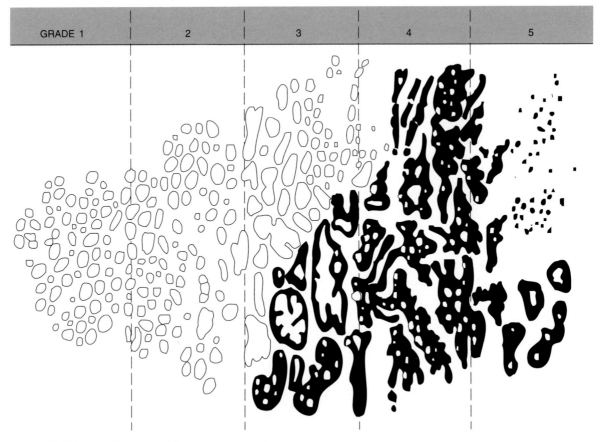

Figure 20 Diagram illustrating Gleason scoring system

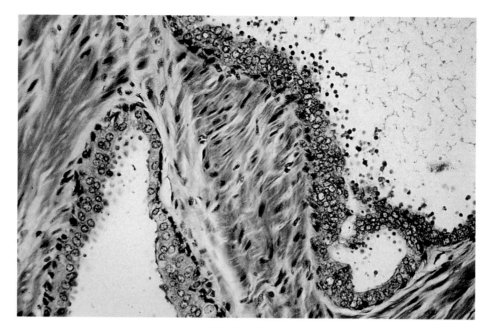

Figure 21 Pathological appearance of high-grade prostatic intraepithelial neoplasia. The luminal epithelium shows loss of polarity, nuclear pleomorphism and nucleoli. The basal cell layer is present and there is no evidence of invasion

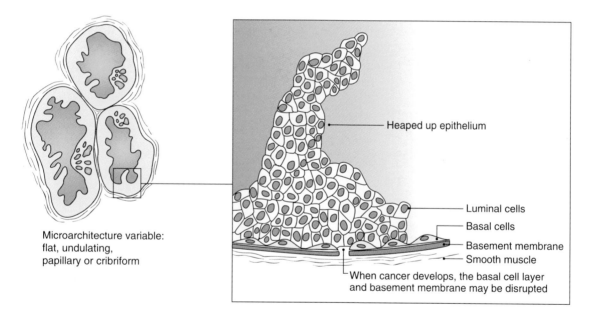

Heaped up epithelium

Luminal cells
Basal cells
Basement membrane
Smooth muscle

When cancer develops, the basal cell layer and basement membrane may be disrupted

Microarchitecture variable: flat, undulating, papillary or cribriform

Figure 22 Diagram demonstrating appearance of high-grade prostatic intraepithelial neoplasia

Watchful waiting

In men beyond the age of 70 and/or significant co-morbidity such as myocardial ischemia or chronic obstructive airways disease, the option of watchful waiting may sometimes be the best course of action. Careful follow-up with regular DRE and PSA monitoring is essential, together with counselling and active involvement of the patient in his own management strategy. Several studies have confirmed that many men whose prostate cancer is managed in this way die with prostate cancer rather than of it.

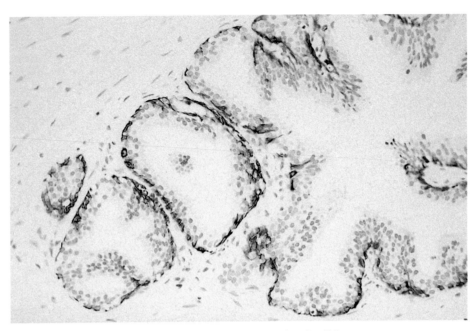

Figure 23 Immunocytochemistry illustrating an intact basal cell layer

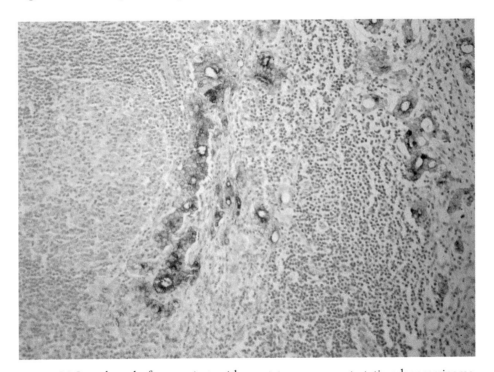

Figure 24 Lymph node from patient with prostate cancer: metastatic adenocarcinoma stains positive for PSA on immunocytochemistry

Radical prostatectomy

Regarded by many as the gold standard therapy, radical prostatectomy has the advantage of not only removing the cancer, but also all other prostate tissue, thereby reducing the likelihood of disease recurrence. The retropubic route is preferred by most urologists; this is accomplished through either a horizontal or vertical skin incision, although a perineal approach is also feasible. Bilateral lymph node sampling is performed, excising the tissue in the triangle lying between the external iliac vein and the obturator nerve (Figure 31a). After division of the endopelvic fascia and both puboprostatic

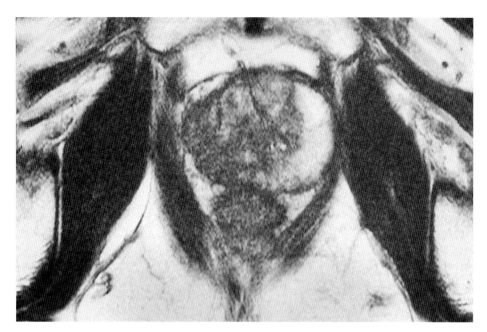

Figure 25 MRI of the prostate showing extraprostatic extension of adenocarcinoma

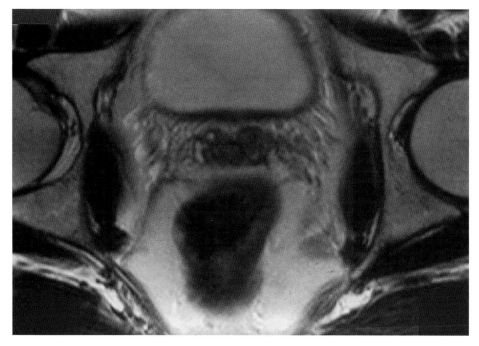

Figure 26 MRI of the prostate showing seminal vesicle infiltration by adenocarcinoma

ligaments, the dorsal venous complex is secured (Figure 31b). The urethra is then divided (Figure 31c), care being taken not to damage the delicate and vulnerable neurovascular bundles lying postero-laterally. Using the divided catheter as a retractor, the lateral pedicles are divided close to the prostate, allowing the neurovascular bundles to displace laterally (Figure 31d). The vasa deferentia are clipped and divided in the mid-line and the seminal vesicles dissected free, care being taken to secure a small artery that usually lies on the medial surface of each structure (Figure 31e). The plane between the prostate and bladder neck is then developed, with careful bladder neck and trigonal preservation. The

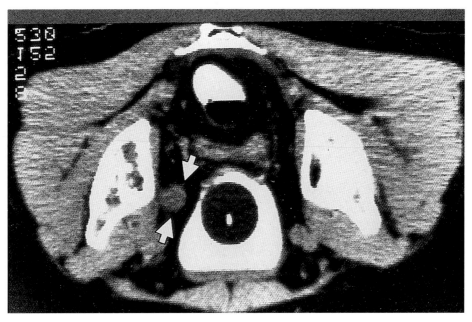

Figure 27 CT scan demonstrating a lymph node (arrowed) involved by prostate carcinoma

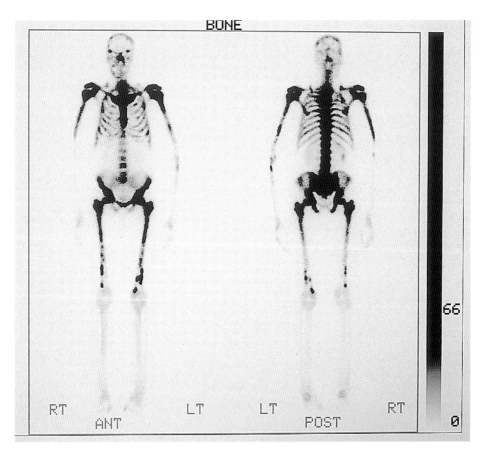

Figure 28 Radionucleide bone scan demonstrating multiple bone metastases due to prostate cancer

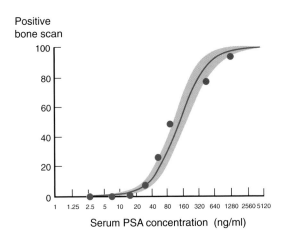

Figure 29 Probability of a positive bone scan for a given PSA value

urethra is then divided at the prostato–vesical junction (Figure 31f). An anastomosis is created between the urethral stump and the bladder neck over a 18 or 20F catheter (Figure 31g). Twin suction wound drains are left down to the pelvis. The prostate, seminal vesicles and lymphatic samples are sent for histological examination. If complete tumor excision has been achieved (Figure 32), the PSA should fall to, and remain at, undetectable levels. Side-effects include erectile dysfunction and (almost always temporary) stress incontinence. Positive surgical margins, especially posterolaterally and at the bladder neck, are associated with a significant risk of local or distant recurrence, as is invasion of the seminal vesicles and especially the discovery of micrometastases in the pelvic lymph nodes. Recently, technological advances have made laparoscopic radical prostatectomy feasible, but few long-term outcome data are yet available.

External beam radiotherapy

External beam radiotherapy (EBRT), often now with conformal imaging (Figure 33), is another frequently employed treatment option for men with clinically localized prostate cancer. No hospitalization is required and a dose of up to 7000 Gy can be administered in divided doses over a 6-week period. One advantage of this treatment option is that pelvic

lymph nodes can also be included in the treatment field. Side-effects include rectal bleeding, hematuria and urinary frequency due to inclusion of the rectum and bladder in the irradiation field. Tumor recurrence cannot usually be treated by surgery; instead, androgen deprivation therapy is generally deployed.

Brachytherapy

Originally popular during the 1960s, brachytherapy has undergone a revival recently as a result of the ability to deploy radioactive seeds accurately under transrectal ultrasound control. Up to 100 seeds, containing either iodine 121 or palladium 103, are placed transperineally into the gland under ultrasound control (Figure 34). Peripheral loading reduces the risk of irradiation damage to the urethra. Results from Seattle suggest that satisfactory long-term PSA reductions can be achieved by this measure, but whether the long-term results are equivalent to surgery or external beam radiotherapy remains currently unclear. In patients considered at high risk of extraprostatic extension of disease, brachytherapy can be combined with EBRT.

Cryotherapy

Cryotherapy to the prostate relies on the use of multiple probes to create an ice-ball involving the gland, with resultant tissue necrosis (Figure 35). Although initially promising results have been reported, others have described a high incidence of side-effects, including pain, urinary retention, erectile dysfunction and occasional fistula formulation. For these reasons, the technique is only occasionally employed and should be regarded as investigational.

Hormonal ablation

Although usually reserved for more advanced prostate tumors, a study is evaluating the use of the antiandrogen bicalutamide in the context of localized disease and has confirmed a significant delay in disease progression (Figure 36) and a highly significant increase in the PSA doubling time. Another place for this form of therapy might be as an adjuvant in patients with positive surgical margins or seminal vesicle involvement after radical prostatectomy, as well as in those patients considered at high risk of relapse after external beam radiotherapy.

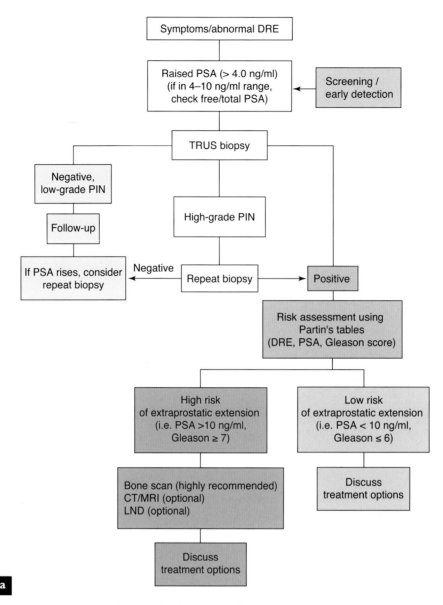

Figure 30 (a) Decision diagram for diagnosis and staging of prostate cancer. DRE, digital rectal examination; PSA, prostate-specific antigen; TRUS, transrectal ultrasound; PIN, prostatic intraepithelial neoplasia; CT, computerized tomography; MRI, magnetic resonance imaging; LND, lymph node dissection

Locally advanced disease

Locally advanced prostate cancer may be defined as extensive cancer that has spread locally beyond the gland to involve the seminal vesicles or bladder neck, but not the lymph nodes or bones (i.e. Stage $T_3N_0M_0$ disease). Rectal examination usually confirms diffuse induration of the gland and the PSA is often > 10 ng/ml. TRUS-guided biopsies confirm extensive infiltration by adenocarcinoma. An MRI scan may reveal distortion of the gland and capsule, with or without seminal vesicle involvement (Figures 26 and 27), but no lymphadenopathy. The bone scan is negative.

Androgen ablation followed by EBRT

The most commonly employed treatment for men with locally advanced prostate cancer is EBRT preceded by androgen ablation (Figure 38). This is

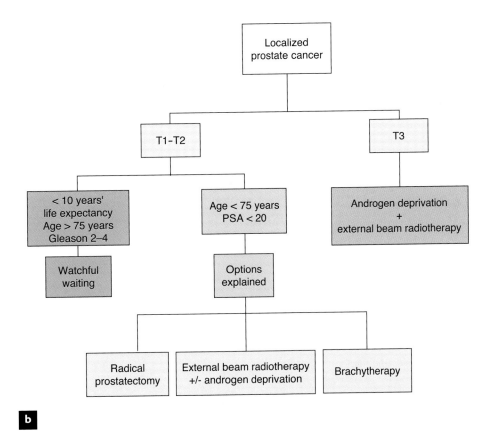

Figure 30 (b) Decision diagram of treatment options for patients with localized prostate cancer

usually achieved by a 3-month depot injection of a luteinizing hormone releasing hormone (LHRH) analog, accompanied for the first 4 weeks by an antiandrogen to prevent tumor flare. EBRT is usually administered daily (excluding weekends) over a 6-week period. Studies by Bolla and colleagues and Pilepich and colleagues have confirmed that both time to progression and overall survival are improved by the combination of androgen ablation with EBRT.

Androgen ablation alone

In older men, and those with pre-existing colorectal disease, androgen ablation alone may be the most appropriate therapy. Androgen ablation can be accomplished most cost-effectively by bilateral orchiectomy; however, most patients prefer non-operative therapy, usually in the form of an LHRH analog administered in three monthly subcutaneous depot injections. Antiandrogens, such as bicalutamide, can also be used in this situation and have the advantage of preserving sexual function. Shortly,

pure LHRH antagonists in the form of the new agent abarelix may also be available for this indication.

Radical surgery preceded by LHRH analogs

Although LHRH analogs have been demonstrated to produce significant gland and tumor shrinkage and consequent reduction of the rate of positive surgical margins, they have not been shown to increase the time to relapse or improve overall survival. At this stage, therefore, this form of treatment should be regarded as investigational rather than standard therapy, although a minority of patients may benefit from such an approach.

Treatment of metastatic disease

In spite of a stage shift in diagnosis of prostate cancer towards earlier disease, a significant proportion of individuals still present with widely disseminated disease. In such circumstances, the PSA is usually markedly elevated. CT or MRI scans usually reveal a T3/T4 lesion in the prostate and associated

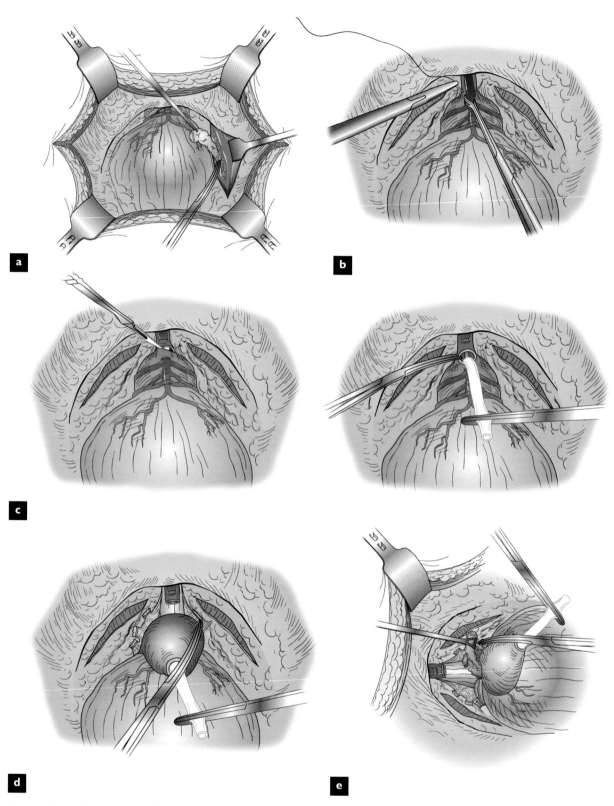

Figure 31 (a) Dissection of obturator lymph nodes; (b) division of the endopelvic fascia and ligation of the dorsal venous complex; (c) division of the urethra; (d) both lateral pedicles are carefully secured, allowing the neurovascular bundles to fall laterally; (e) both vasa deferentia are divided and the seminal vesicles dissected free, carefully controlling the blood vessels that usually run up their medial surface

Continued

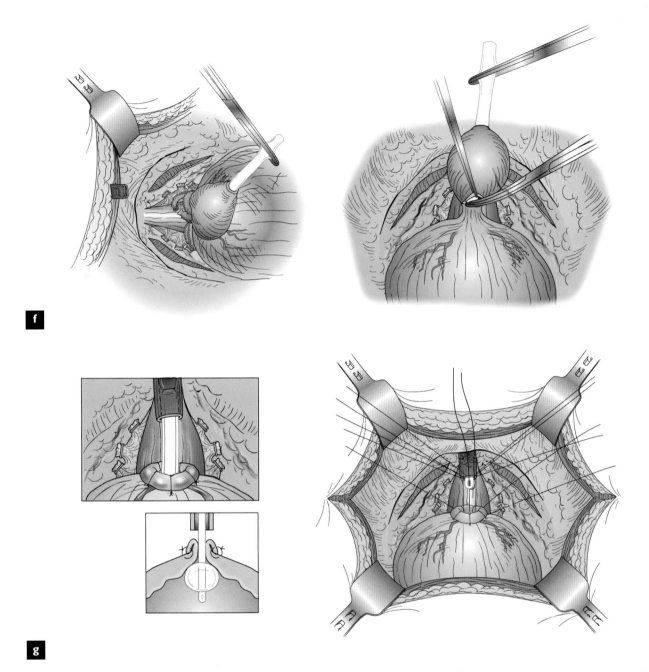

Figure 31 (*continued*) (f) The bladder neck is preserved as the prostate is dissected away; (g) an anastomosis is created between the urethra and the bladder neck

lymphadenopathy. A bone scan is often positive. Metastatic prostate can also develop after failed attempts at curative therapy. Patients with positive surgical margins (Figure 39) or cancer outside the prostate (Figure 40) are particularly at risk.

First-line treatment for metastatic prostate cancer is androgen deprivation. This can be achieved by bilateral orchiectomy (Figure 41). Because of the reluctance of men to undergo castration, the most frequently employed treatment is the administration of LHRH analogs (Figure 42). These act as super-agonists on LHRH receptors in the pituitary, first overstimulating them and eventually (after around 2 weeks) blocking the release of luteinizing hormone, thereby reducing circulating testosterone levels to castrate values. Prior to their administration, it is wise to administer an antiandrogen, such as bicalu-tamide, to prevent the so-called 'tumor flare'

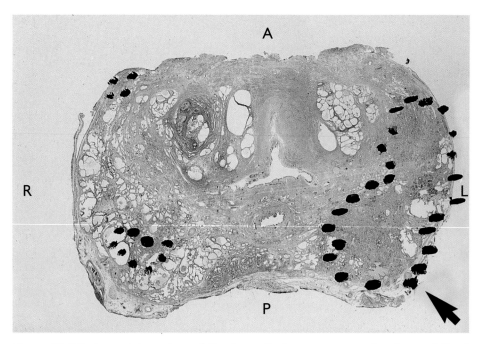

Figure 32 Whole mount specimen following radical prostatectomy showing multifocal prostate cancer, which is specimen-confined. In large series of radical prostatectomies, an average of 3.5 separate cancers were found in each specimen

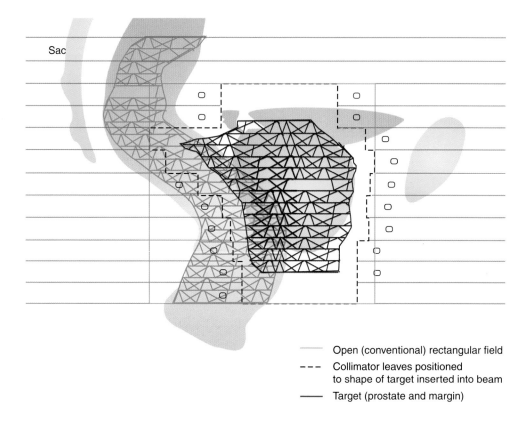

—— Open (conventional) rectangular field

- - - Collimator leaves positioned to shape of target inserted into beam

—— Target (prostate and margin)

Figure 33 Conformal radiotherapy allows more accurate targeting of the radiation dosage to the prostate

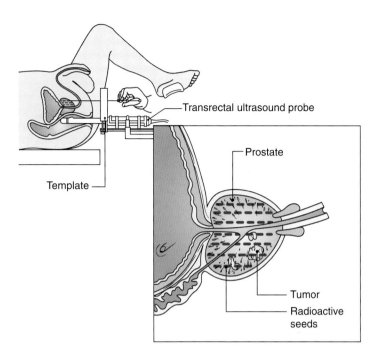

Figure 34 Brachytherapy for adenocarcinoma showing technique of seed insertion

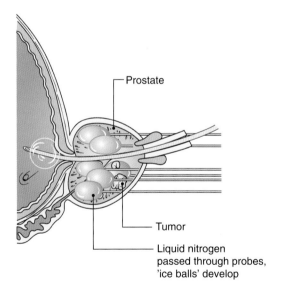

Figure 35 Cryotherapy

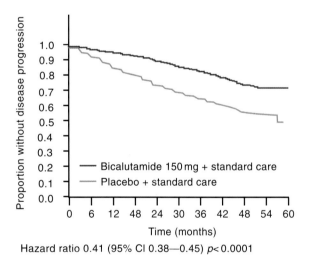

Hazard ratio 0.41 (95% CI 0.38—0.45) *p*< 0.0001

Figure 36 Effect of bicalutamide in delaying prostate cancer progression

response to the initial increase in circulating serum testosterone, which can occasionally result in spinal cord compression. These are usually continued for 4–6 weeks, although some clinicians prescribe antiandrogens and LHRH analogs in combination in the longer term. The rationale for the latter

approach is that adrenal androgens are not suppressed by LHRH analogs but are blocked by antiandrogens (Figure 43). Data are currently conflicting as to whether this 'combined androgen blockade' (CAB) significantly increases the time to progression or overall survival.

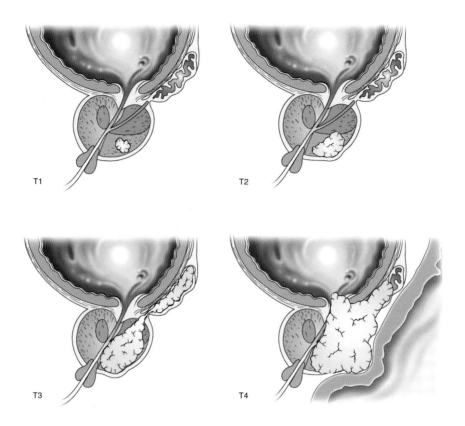

Figure 37 Local staging of prostate cancer

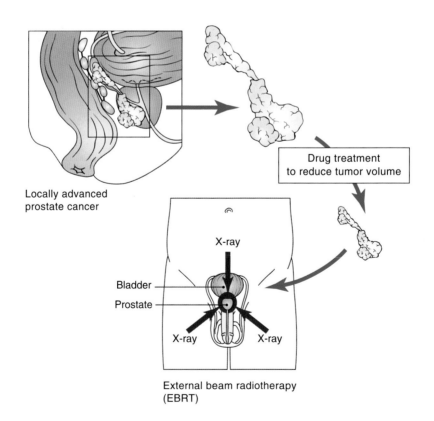

Figure 38 Locally advanced prostate cancer: hormonal therapy followed by external beam radiotherapy

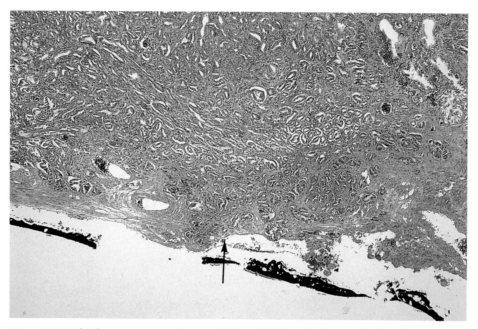

Figure 39 Radical prostatectomy histopathology: the limit has been inked. A focal positive surgical margin is present

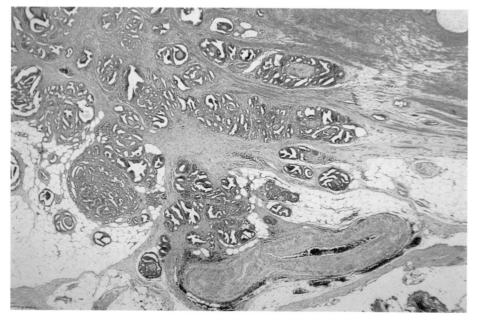

Figure 40 Radical prostatectomy histopathology showing extraprostatic extension of adenocarcinoma associated with a fibrous response

Recently, a new treatment option for metastatic prostate cancer has been developed, namely an LHRH agonist, known as abarelix. This offers the potential advantage of more rapid achievement of castrate levels of testosterone and avoids the risks of tumor flare. As a consequence, there will be no need to administer antiandrogens concomitantly with this form of therapy.

MANAGEMENT OF HORMONE-ESCAPED PROSTATE CANCER

Presumably by a process of clonal selection, almost all locally advanced and metastatic prostate cancers eventually become insensitive to androgen ablation and demonstrate the phenomenon known as 'hormone escape' (Figure 44). A number of

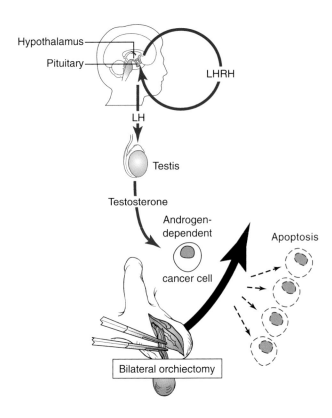

Figure 41 Bilateral orchiectomy results in apoptosis of cancer cells and disease remission

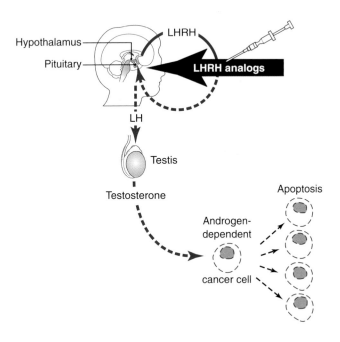

Figure 42 LHRH analog therapy produces a result equivalent to orchiectomy

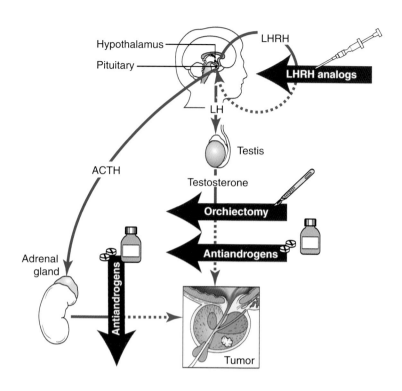

Figure 43 Maximum androgen blockade prevents stimulation of the tumor, not only by testosterone but also by adrenal androgens

mechanisms, including mutations involving the androgen receptor, have been proposed as the cause. The consequence is that, after a variable period of PSA suppression, serum levels of this marker eventually begin to rise. This PSA increase usually heralds clinical symptoms – often the development of bone pain or less commonly spinal cord compression (Figure 45), with an average lag of 8–12 months.

At the time of a PSA increase, in spite of endocrine ablation, restaging of the disease with a bone scan may be indicated. Of more importance to the patient, however, is which therapeutic maneuver should be made. If the patient is being treated with an antiandrogen, such as bicalutamide or flutamide, this should usually be stopped. Antiandrogen withdrawal alone may result in a temporary PSA decline. The explanation for this antiandrogen insensitivity is still debated, but it may be the result of alterations in androgen receptors so that former antagonists act as agonists and actually stimulate prostate cancer cell growth. A similar phenomenon has been observed with antiestrogens, such as tamoxifen, in breast cancer.

A second move is to add an estrogen, usually stilbestrol at either 1 or 3 mg/day or estracyt. Estrogens appear to exert a direct cytotoxic effect on prostate cancer cells and may induce a second response, which is occasionally quite durable. Because of their well-recognized thromboembolic properties, it is wise to use them in conjunction with aspirin at a dose of 75–150 mg/day, providing there are no gastrointestinal contraindications. During this treatment, those patients on LHRH analogs/antagonists should be continued on this, because any rise in serum testosterone is only likely to result in even faster clinical deterioration.

A further maneuver that has been found to be effective in some patients is to use chemotherapy with agents such as mitozantrone or taxotere, or add in a steroid such as hydrocortisone, although the mechanism for the effect of steroids in this situation is not entirely clear. If pain is localized to a specific area (lower back or pelvis, for example), then a short course of radiotherapy may be helpful. If the pain from bone metastases is multifocal, a single administration of strontium has been shown to be beneficial.

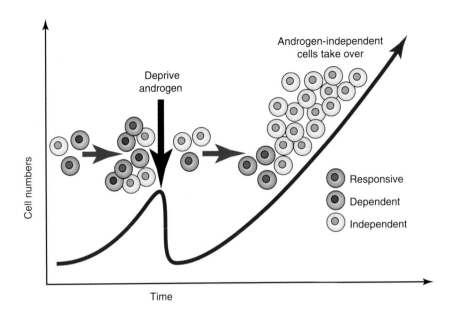

Figure 44 Development of androgen independence due to the proliferation of androgen-insensitive cells

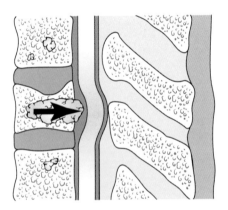

Figure 45 Spinal cord compression due to metastatic prostate cancer

What are needed urgently are new agents that have efficacy and acceptable tolerability in patients with a rising PSA, in spite of androgen ablation therapy and/or estrogens. A number of promising agents are currently being investigated, including tyrosine kinase inhibitors, endothelin antagonists and anti-angiogenesis agents. The results of randomized controlled trials will be needed to confirm their safety and efficacy.

FURTHER READING

Adolfsson J, Steineck G, Hediund PO. Deferred treatment of locally advanced nonmetastatic prostate cancer: a long-term follow-up. *J Urol* 1999;161:505–8

Anscher J, Clough R, Dodge R. Radiotherapy for a rising prostate-specific antigen after radical prostatectomy: the first 10 years. *Int J Radiat Oncol Biol Phys* 2000;48:369–75

Blute ML, Bergstralh EJ, Partin AW, *et al.* Validation of Partin tables for predicting pathological stage of clinically localized prostate cancer. *J Urol* 2000:164:1591–5

Becker C, Piironen T, Pettersson K, *et al.* Clinical value of human glandular kallikrein 2 and free and total prostate-specific antigen in serum from a population of men with prostate-specific antigen levels 3.0 ng/mL or greater. *Urology* 2000;55:694–9

Bolla M, Gonzalez D, Warde P, *et al.* Improved survival in patients with locally advanced prostate cancer treated with radiotherapy and goserelin. *N Engl J Med* 1997;337:295–300

Brawer MK. Prostate-specific antigen: current status. *CA Cancer J Clin* 1999;49:264–81

Brawer MK, Cheli CD, Neaman IE, *et al.* Complexed PSA specificity in detecting CPA. *J Urol* 2000;163:1476–9

Catalona WF, Ramos CG, Carvalhal GF. Contemporary results of anatomic radical prostatectomy. *CA Cancer J Clin* 1999;49:282–96

Crawford ED. Combined androgen blockade. *Eur Urol* 1996;29(Suppl 2):54–61

D'Amico AV, Schultz D, Loffredo M, *et al.* Biochemical outcome following external beam radiation therapy with or without androgen suppression therapy for clinically localized prostate cancer. *J Am Med Assoc* 2000;284:1280–3

D'Amico AV, Whittington R, Malkowicz SB, *et al.* Clinical utility of the percentage of positive prostate biopsies in defining biochemical outcome after radical prostatectomy for patients with clinically localized prostate cancer. *J Clin Oncol* 2000;18:1164–72

Davis JW, Kolm P, Wright Jr GL, *et al.* The durability of external beam radiation therapy for prostate cancer: can it be identified? *J Urol* 1999;162:758–61

de la Taille A, Hayek O, Benson MC, *et al.* Salvage cryotherapy for recurrent prostate cancer after radiation therapy: the Columbia experience. *Urology* 2000;55:79–84

Gage AA, Huben RR. Cryosurgical ablation of the prostate. *Urol Oncol* 1999;5:11–19

Goode EL, Stanford JL, Chakrabarti L, *et al.* Linkage analysis of 150 high-risk prostate cancer families at 1 q24-25. *Genet Epidemiol* 2000;18:251–75

Grimm PD, Blasko JC, Ragde E, *et al.* Does brachytherapy have a role in the treatment of prostate cancer. *Hematol Oncol Clin North Am* 1996;10:653–73

Hanks G. Conformal radiotherapy for prostate cancer. *Ann Med* 2000;32:57–63

Haese A, Becker C, Noldus J, *et al.* Human glandular kallikrein 2: a potential serum marker for predicting the organ confined versus non-organ confined growth of prostate cancer. *J Urol* 2000;163:1491–7

Kahn D, Williams RD, Haseman MK, Reed NL, Miller SJ, Gerstbrein JJ. Radioimmunoscintigraphy with In-111-labeled capromab pendetide predicts prostate cancer response to salvage radiotherapy after failed radical prostatectomy. *J Clin Oncol* 1998;16:284–9

Kim ED, Scardino PT, Hampel O, *et al.* Interposition of sural nerve restores function of cavernous nerves resected during radical prostatectomy. *J Urol* 1999;161:188–92

Kirby RS. Treatment options for early prostate cancer. *Urology* 1998;52:948–62

Kirby RS. Pre-treatment staging of prostate cancer: recent advances and future prospects. *Prostate Cancer and Prostatic Diseases* 1997;1:2–10

Klotz L. Neurostimulation during radical prostatectomy: improving nerve-sparing techniques. *Semin Urol Oncol* 2000;18:46–50

Koppie TM, Shinohara K, Grossfeld GD, *et al.* The efficacy of cryosurgical ablation of prostate cancer: the University of California, San Francisco experience. *J Urol* 1999;162:427–32

Lee CT, Fair WR. The role of dietary manipulation in biochemical recurrence of prostate cancer after radical prostatectomy. *Semin Urol Oncol* 1999;17:154–63

Manyak MJ, Javitt MC. The role of computerized tomography, magnetic resonance imaging, bone scan, and mono-clonal antibody nuclear scan for prognosis prediction in prostate cancer. *Semin Urol Oncol* 1998;16:145–52

Messing EM, Manola J, Sarsosdy M, *et al.* Immediate hormonal therapy compared with observation after radical prostatectomy and pelvic lymphadenectomy in men with node positive prostate cancer. *N Engl J Med* 1999;341:1781–8

Mettlin C, Murphy GP. Why is the prostate cancer death rate declining in the United States? *Cancer* 1998;82:249–51

Monk T, Goddnough LT, Brecher ME, *et al.* A prospective randomized comparison of three blood conservation strategies for radical prostatectomy. *Anesthesiology* 1999;91:24–33

Montie JE, Wei JT. Artificial neural networks for prostate carcinoma risk assessment. *Cancer* 2000;88:2655–60

Nag S, Fernandes PS, Bahnson R. Transperineal image-guided permanent brachytherapy for localized cancer of the prostate. *Urol Oncol* 1998;4:191–202

Olsson CA, de Vries GM, Buttyan R, Katz AE. Reverse transcriptase-polymerase chain reaction assays for prostate cancer. *Urol Clin North Am* 1997;24:367–78

Pannek J, Partin AW. The role of PSA and percent free PSA for staging and prognosis prediction in clinically localized prostate cancer. *Semin Urol Oncol* 1998;16:100–5

Partin AW, Kattan MW, Subong ENP, *et al.* Combination of prostate-specific antigen, clinical stage and Gleason score to predict pathological stage of localized prostate cancer. *J Am Med Assoc* 1997;277:1445–51

Polascik TI, Pond CR, DeWeese TL, Walsh PC. Comparison of radical prostatectomy and iodine 125 inter-stitial radiotherapy for the treatment of clinically localized prostate cancer: a 7 year biochemical (PSA) progression analysis. *Urology* 1998;51:884–90

Potters L, Torre T, Ashley R, Leibel S. Examining the role of neoadjuvant androgen deprivation in patients undergoing prostate brachytherapy. *J Clin Oncol* 2000;18:1187–92

Pound CR, Partin AW, Eisenberger MA, *et al.* Natural history of progression after PSA elevation following radical prostatectomy. *J Am Med Assoc* 1999;281:1591–7

Prestidge BR, Prete JJ, Buchholz TA, *et al.* A survey of current clinical practice of permanent prostate brachytherapy in the United States. *Physics* 1998;40:461

Ragde H, Eigamal AA, Snow PB, *et al.* Ten-year disease free survival after transperineal sonography-guided iodine-125 brachytherapy with or without 45-gray external beam irradiation in the treatment of patients with clinically localized, low to high Gleason grade prostate carcinoma. *Cancer* 1998;83:989–1001

Ragde H, Korb LJ, Eigamat AA, *et al.* Modern prostate brachytherapy. *Cancer* 2000;89:135–41

Ramos CG, Carvalhal GF, Smith DS, *et al.* Retrospective comparison of radical retropubic prostatectomy and 125iodine brachytherapy for localized prostate cancer. *J Urol* 1999;161:1212–15

Rehman J, Christ GJ, Kaynan A, *et al.* Intraoperative electrical stimulation of cavernosal nerves with monitoring of intracorporeal pressure in patient undergoing nerve sparing radical prostatectomy. *Br J Urol Int* 1999;84: 305–10

Richert-Boe KE, Humphrey LL, Glass AG, *et al.* Screening digital rectal examination and prostate cancer mortality: a case control study. *J Med Screen* 1998;5:99–103

Roberts RO, Bergstrath EJ, Katusic SK, *et al.* Decline in prostate cancer mortality from 1980 to 1997, and an update on incidence trends in Olmstead County, Minnesota. *J Urol* 1999;161:529–33

Robinson JW, Saliken JC, Donnelly BJ, *et al.* Quality-of-life outcomes for men treated with cryosurgery for localized prostate carcinoma. *Cancer* 1999;86:1793–801

Schmidt JD, Doyle J, Larison S. Prostate cryoablation: update 1998. *CA Cancer J Clin* 1998;48:239

Scolieri MJ, Aftman A, Resnick MI. Neoadjuvant androgen deprivation prior to radical prostatectomy. *J Urol* 2000;164:1465–70

Seay TM, Blute ML, Zincke H. Long-term outcome in patients with pTxN+ adenocarcinoma of prostate treated with radical prostatectomy and early androgen ablation. *J Urol* 1998;159:357

Sharkey J, Chovnick SD, Behar Ri, *et al.* Outpatient ultrasound-guided palladium 103 brachytherapy for localized adenocarcinoma of the prostate: a preliminary report of 434 patients. *Urology* 1998;51:796

Shipley WU, Thames HD, Sandler HM, *et al.* Radiation therapy for clinically localized prostate cancer: a multi-institutional pooled analysis. *J Am Med Assoc* 1999;281:1598–604

Stanford JL, Feng Z, Hamilton AS, *et al.* Urinary and sexual function after radical prostatectomy for clinically localized prostate cancer. *J Am Med Assoc* 2000;283:354–60

Stock RG, Stone NN. Permanent radioactive seed implantation in the treatment of prostate cancer. *Hem Onc Clin N Am* 1999;13:489–501

Vassilikos EJ, Yu H, Trochtenburg J, *et al.* Relapse and cure rates of prostate cancer patients after radical prostatectomy and 5 years of follow-up. *Clin Biochem* 2000;33:115–23

Vicini FA, Kini R, Edmundson G, *et al.* A comprehensive review of prostate cancer brachytherapy: defining an optimal technique. *Int J Radiat Oncol Biol Phys* 1999;44:483–91

Visakorpi T. Molecular genetics of prostate cancer. *Ann Chir Gynaecol* 1999;88:11–16

Walsh PC, Marschke P, Ricker D, Burnett AL. Patient-reported urinary continence and sexual function after anatomic radical prostatectomy. *Urology* 2000;55:58–61

Wieder JA, Soloway MS. Incidence, etiology, location, prevention and treatment of positive surgical margins after radical prostatectomy for prostate cancer. *J Urol* 1998;160:299

Wilder RB, Hsiang JY, Ji M, *et al.* Preliminary results of three-dimensional conformal radiotherapy as salvage treatment for a rising prostate-specific antigen level postprostatectomy. *Am J Clin Oncol* 2000;23:176–80

Wilson MJ. Prostate-specific antigen (hK3) and human prostatic glandular kallikrein (hK2) in the detection of early stage human prostate cancer. *J Lab Clin Med* 1998;131:298

Wirth M, Tyrell C, Wallace M, *et al.* Bicalutamide (Casodex) 150 mg as immediate therapy in patients with localized or locally advanced prostate cancer significantly reduces the risk of progression. *Urology* 2001;58:146–51

Yoshida BA, Chekmareva MA, Wharam JF, *et al.* Prostate cancer metastasis-suppressor genes: a current perspective. *In Vivo* 1998;12:49–58

Young CY, Seay T, Hogen K, *et al.* Prostate-specific human kallikrein (hK2) as a novel marker for prostate cancer. *Prostate* 1996;7(Suppl):17–24

3

Renal cancer

Adenocarcinoma of the kidney is an important urological malignancy, but one that is much less prevalent than prostate cancer. It is a disease that predominantly affects middle-aged and elderly people, with a slight male to female preponderance. Occasionally, cases are seen in younger adults. The tumor probably arises from the epithelial cell component of the renal tubules and results in a characteristic 'clear cell' histological pattern of differing degrees of differentiation (Figure 46). Most cases are sporadic, but a small number are hereditary – usually in association with the Von Hippel–Lindau syndrome.

DIAGNOSIS

The classical triad with which a renal cancer presents, namely an abdominal mass, loin discomfort and hematuria, is much less frequently encountered now. Increasingly, renal tumors are diagnosed as 'incidentalomas' during scanning of the abdomen and retroperitoneum for a variety of reasons. Any patient with unexplained hematuria should be investigated to rule out a renal tumor as a cause of the bleeding. An intravenous urogram (Figure 47) may reveal irregularity of the renal outline or distortion of the calyceal anatomy. An ultrasound study will confirm the presence of a solid, space-occupying lesion (Figure 48), and can distinguish it from a much more commonly encountered benign renal cyst. CT scanning (Figure 49) and MRI (Figure 50) can be helpful in staging the tumor or tumors. In atypical cases, where lymphoma or other pathology is suspected, an ultrasound- or CT-guided biopsy may be indicated.

STAGING

The staging of renal adenocarcinoma is demonstrated in Figure 51. Local extension can occur to perinephric fat and adjacent structures. This tumor has a pronounced tendency to extend into the renal vein. From there, involvement of the inferior vena cava and even extension into the right atrium may occur. Renal ultrasound will usually identify involvement of the renal vein or inferior vena cava, but a contrast study of the inferior vena cava itself is often required to delineate its upper extent. An MRI or

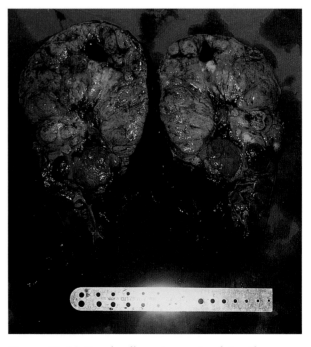

Figure 46 (a) Renal cell carcinoma involving the upper pole of the kidney

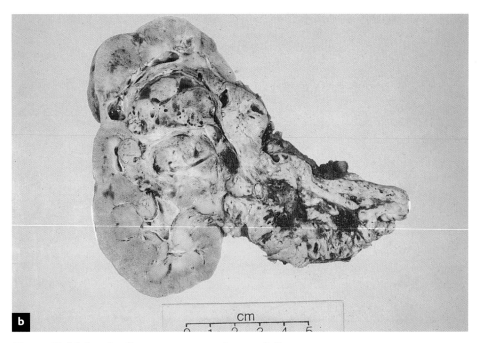

Figure 46 (b) Renal cell carcinoma extending medially

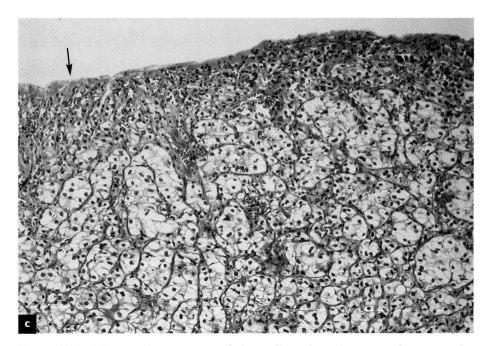

Figure 46 (c) Microscopic appearance of clear cell renal carcinoma invading up to the pelvic urothelium (arrow)

spiral CT can also be of assistance in this context (Figure 52).

More distant spread occurs predominantly to the local lymph nodes, lungs and other soft tissues (Figure 53). Bone metastases may also occur, causing local swelling and pain, or pathological fractures.

TREATMENT

Notwithstanding recent advances in our understanding of the genetics and biology of renal cell carcinoma, surgery remains the cornerstone of curative treatment for this disease (see decision diagram,

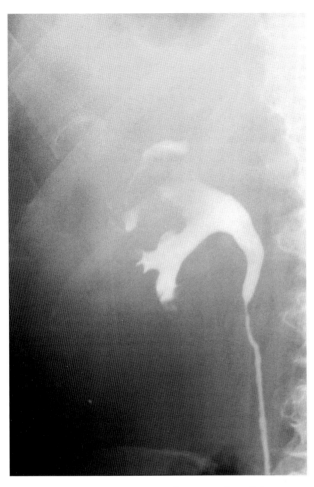

Figure 47 Intravenous urogram showing calyceal distortion due to renal cell carcinoma

Figure 54). Nonetheless, the role of surgery is evolving with respect to both localized renal cell carcinoma and in patients who present with metastatic disease. Nephron-sparing surgery is assuming an increasingly important role in the management of localized tumors. The advent of promising immunotherapy and other new disease management strategies, including gene therapy, used in an adjunctive role with surgery is beginning to offer new hope for those unfortunate patients with disseminated malignancy.

RADICAL NEPHRECTOMY

Radical nephrectomy was established as the gold-standard, curative operation for localized renal cell carcinoma by Robson and colleagues with their report of 66% and 64% overall survival of patients with stage I and stage II tumors. These results were superior to those achieved in patients undergoing simple pericapsular nephrectomy. More recent reports have indicated more than 80% survival following radical nephrectomy for stage I (T1–T2) renal cell carcinoma.

Radical nephrectomy (Figure 55) necessitates early identification and ligation of the renal artery and vein, removal of the kidney and perinephric fat, outside Gerota's fascia, excision of the ipsilateral

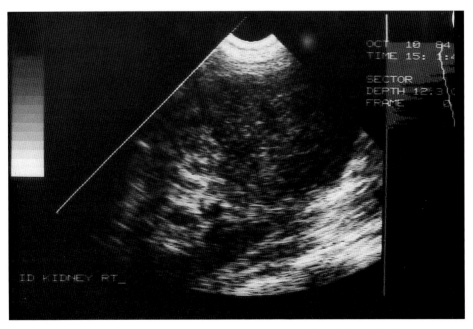

Figure 48 Ultrasound showing the echodense appearance of a solid renal cell carcinoma

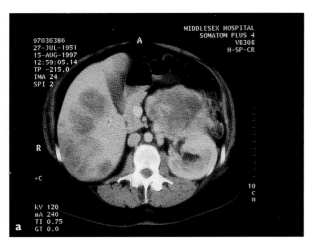 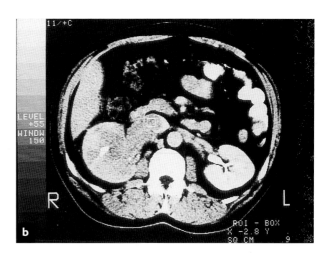

Figure 49 CT scan demonstrating (a) a large left renal cell carcinoma and (b) a tumor with right renal vein involvement

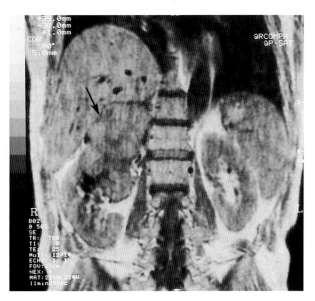

Figure 50 MRI showing a right-sided renal cell carcinoma in the upper pole of the kidney (arrowed)

adrenal gland and the performance of a regional lymphadenectomy. In recent years, the need for so radical an approach in every patient has been questioned. Performance of the perifascial nephrectomy is of undoubted importance in preventing local tumor recurrence, because approximately 25% of localized renal cell carcinomas will manifest perinephric fat involvement. Preliminary renal artery ligation remains an accepted practice; however, in large tumors with abundant collateral vascular supply, it is not always possible to achieve complete initial control of the arterial circulation. It has now been clearly demonstrated that it is not always necessary to remove the ipsilateral adrenal gland, unless the adjacent upper portion of the

kidney is involved with renal cell carcinoma. The need for extensive lymphadenectomy is currently unproven, although a subset of patients with micrometastases may conceivably benefit. The procedure does add to the complexity of the operation and carries with it a small but significant risk of morbidity, usually from postoperative bleeding, and should therefore probably be confined to those cases felt to be at particular risk of lymph node involvement. Laparoscopic nephrectomy is now increasingly being employed for smaller tumors and may soon become the standard of care (Figure 56).

NEPHRON-SPARING SURGERY

Partial nephrectomy or 'nephron-sparing surgery' has become an increasingly successful form of treatment for patients with localized renal cell carcinoma in whom there is a need to preserve functioning renal parenchyma. Accepted indications include situations in which radical nephrectomy would render the patient anephric, with a subsequent immediate need for dialysis. This includes individuals with either bilateral renal cell carcinoma or renal cell carcinoma in a solitary kidney. The latter circumstance may be the result of unilateral renal agenesis, previous removal of the contralateral kidney or irreversible impairment of contralateral kidney function.

Another indication for nephron-sparing surgery is a patient with unilateral renal cell carcinoma and a functioning opposite kidney that is threatened with future impairment. Examples include renal artery stenosis, chronic pyelonephritis, stone disease or systemic disorders such as diabetes mellitus.

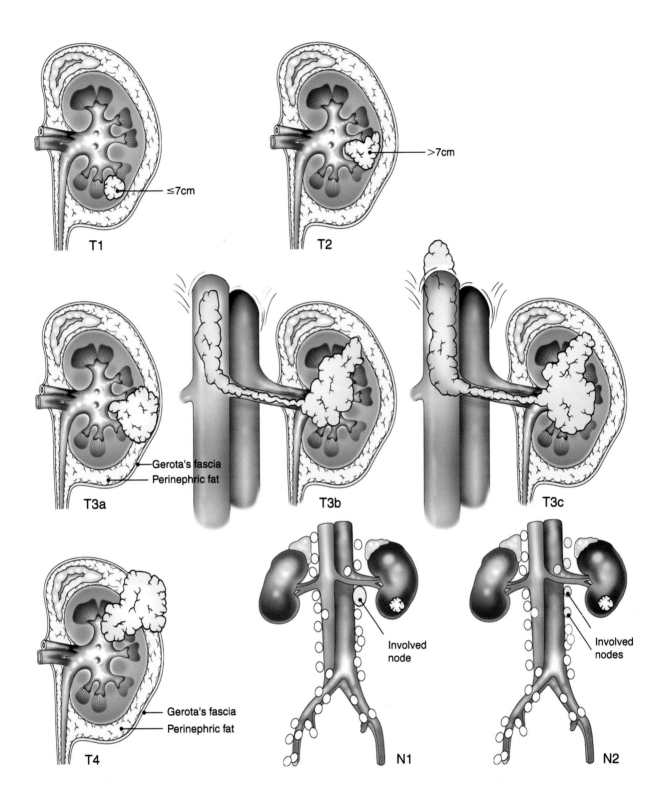

Figure 51 Staging diagram for renal cell carcinoma

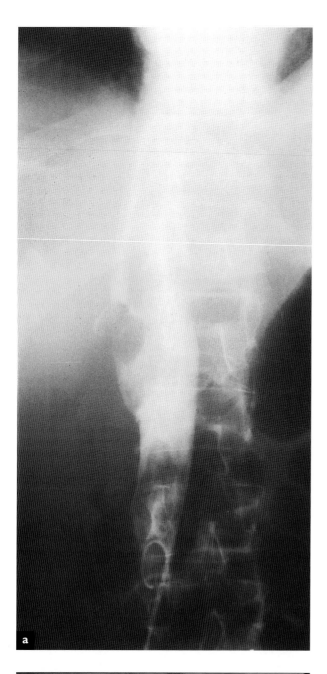

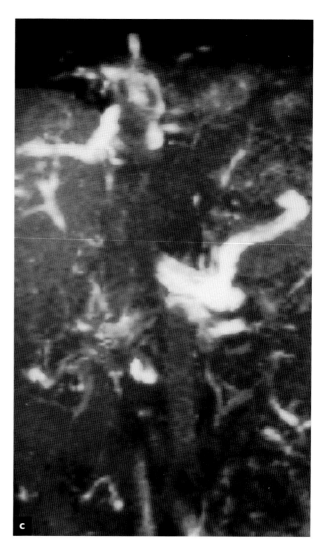

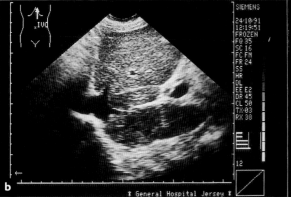

Figure 52 Renal cell carcinoma: IVC involvement (a) cavagram (b) ultrasound (c) MRI

OPERATIVE TECHNIQUE FOR PARTIAL NEPHRECTOMY

Before radical nephrectomy, preoperative arteriography to delineate intrarenal vasculature is usually unnecessary. However, if partial nephrectomy is being considered, then this information may facilitate both the planning and execution of the procedure. It is usually possible to perform partial nephrectomy for renal cell carcinoma *in situ* by using an operative technique that combines optimal exposure of the kidney with an understanding of the renal vascular anatomy in relation to the tumor. An extraperitoneal flank incision through the bed of the 10th or 11th rib is employed for almost all of these procedures. Occasionally, a thoraco-abdominal incision is required for very large tumors that involve the upper portion of the kidney. By comparison, an anterior subcostal approach results in the kidney being

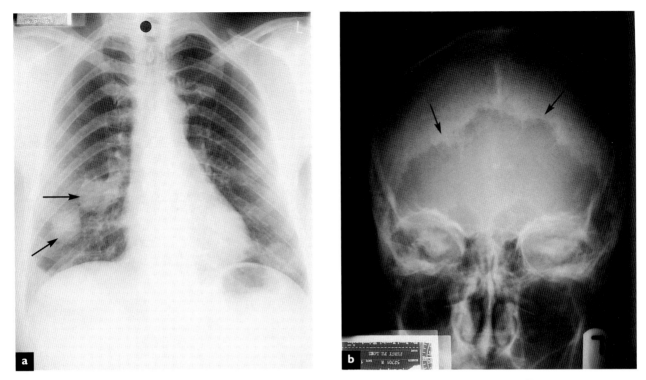

Figure 53 (a) Multiple pulmonary metastases; (b) skull X-ray showing bone metastasis from renal cell carcinoma

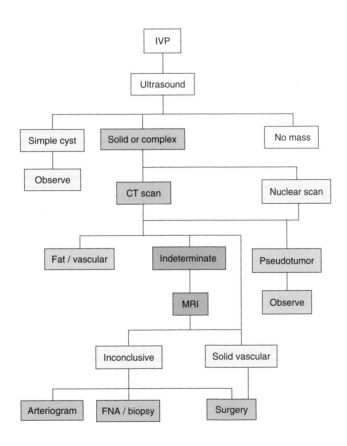

Figure 54 (a) Evaluation of a renal mass. IVP, intravenous pyelogram; CT, computerized tomography; MRI, magnetic resonance imaging; FNA, fine needle aspiration

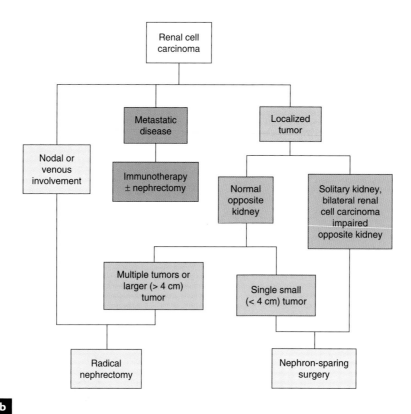

Figure 54 (b) Decision diagram illustrating the diagnosis and management of renal cell carcinoma

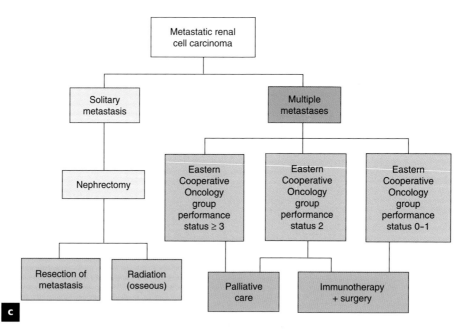

Figure 54 (c) Decision diagram illustrating the diagnosis and management of metastatic renal cell carcinoma

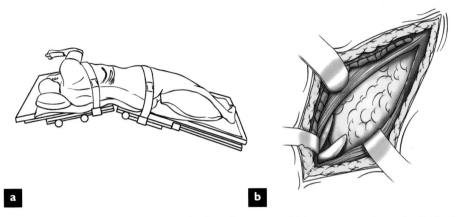

Figure 55 (a) Patient position for radical nephrectomy; (b) loin incision above the 12th rib

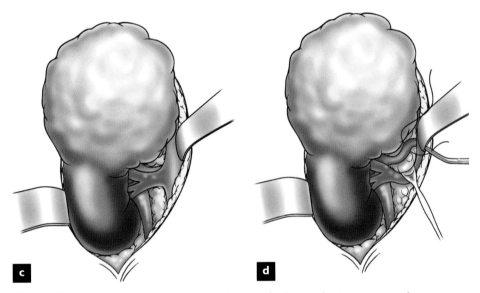

Figure 55 (c) Exposure of renal artery and vein; (d) the renal artery is secured

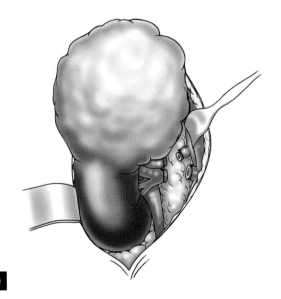

Figure 55 (e) Ligation and division of renal vein

located in the depths of the wound, and the surgical exposure is simply not as good.

The kidney is mobilized within Gerota's fascia, leaving the perinephric fat around the tumor itself (Figure 57). For small peripheral tumors, it may not be necessary to control the renal artery. In most cases, however, partial nephrectomy is most effectively performed after temporary renal arterial occlusion. In most cases, it is important to have the renal vein patent throughout the operation.

While the renal circulation is temporarily occluded *in situ*, renal hypothermia is used to protect against ischemic renal injury. Surface cooling of the kidney with ice slush allows up to 3 hours of safe ischaemia without permanent renal injury. Several surgical techniques are available for *in situ* partial

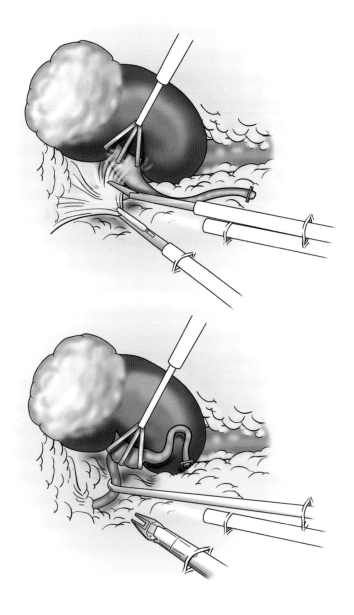

Figure 56 Laparoscopic nephrectomy: the ureter is divided before the renal artery and vein are secured and removal of the kidney

nephrectomy for patients with renal cell carcinoma. These include polar segmental excision, wedge resection and transverse resection. All of those techniques require adherence to basic principles of early vascular control, avoidance of ischemic renal damage, complete tumor excision with uninvolved surgical margins, precise closure of the collecting system and careful hemostasis.

Partial nephrectomy carries a higher operative and postoperative morbidity than radical nephrec-

tomy. The most common serious complications are urinary fistula formation and acute renal failure. In most cases, renal failure resolves spontaneously, but occasionally (about 4% of cases) this may be permanent and patients should be pre-informed accordingly. One potential disadvantage of partial nephrectomy for renal cell carcinoma is the risk of local recurrence on the operated kidney, which has been observed in 4–6% of cases. Careful follow-up is therefore required.

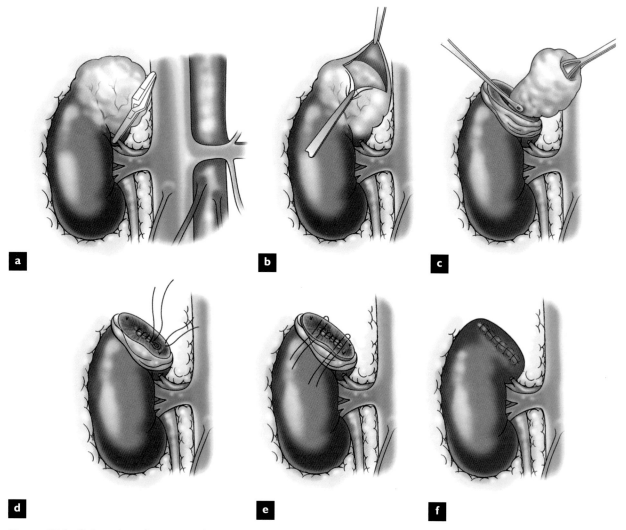

Figure 57 (a–f) Partial nephrectomy: the arterial supply to the upper renal segment is clamped temporarily. The involved segment is removed and the defect repaired

RENAL CELL CARCINOMA WITH VENA CAVA INVOLVEMENT

One of the unique features of renal cell carcinoma is its pronounced tendency to grow intraluminally within the renal venous circulation. For patients with non-metastatic renal cell carcinoma and inferior vena cava involvement, 5-year survival rates of 47–68% have been reported following complete surgical excision. The presence of either lymph node or distant metastases in such cases carries a dismal prognosis that is not influenced by surgical extirpation.

When undertaking surgical removal of a tumor thrombus in the inferior vena cava, it is essential to obtain control of the vena cava above the thrombus to prevent intraoperative embolization of tumor fragment (Figure 58). Temporary occlusion of the infrahepatic inferior vena cava can safely be performed, but occlusion of the supradiaphragmatic inferior vena cava often causes a profound decrease in venous return, with consequent hypotension. Although techniques such as intrapericardial clamping of the inferior vena cava with simultaneous occlusion of the porta hepatis and superior mesenteric artery have been described, cardiopulmonary bypass with deep hypothermic circulatory arrest has some advantages, but mortality rates of 4.5–13% have been reported.

MANAGEMENT OF METASTATIC DISEASE

Altogether, around one-third of all patients with renal cell carcinoma present with established metastases – often diagnosed on chest X-ray (Figure 53a). A further 30–40% of the remainder will eventually develop metastases in spite of best efforts to excise the primary tumor.

Until recently, there were relatively few indications for surgery in patients with metastatic renal cell carcinoma. The incidence of spontaneous regression of metastatic renal cell carcinoma after removal of

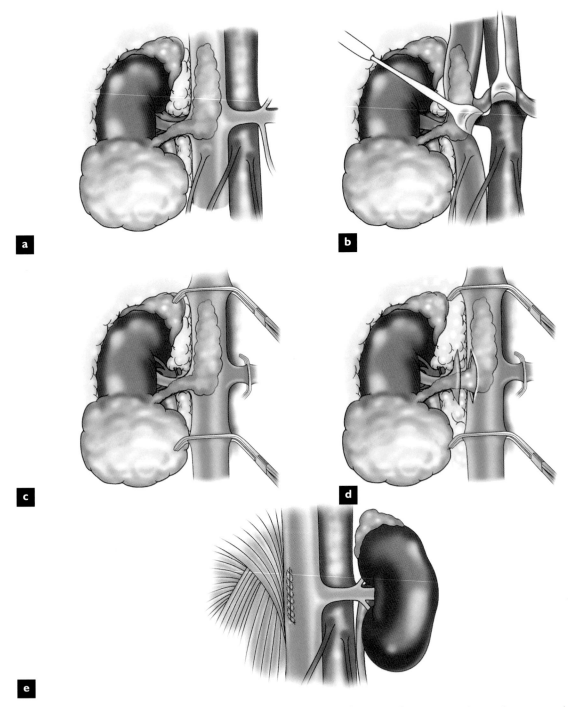

Figure 58 Inferior vena cava involvement: surgical approach to achieve nephrectomy and complete removal of the tumor thrombus. (a) The kidney and great vessels are exposed; (b) the renal artery is secured; (c) the inferior vena cava is controlled; (d) the kidney is removed and the tumor thrombus gently extracted from the inferior vena cava; (e) the inferior vena cava is repaired

the primary tumor is only in the order of 1–4% and, therefore, nephrectomy on this basis is no longer justified. There is a palliative role for nephrectomy in selected patients with metastatic renal cell carcinoma who are experiencing severe disability from local associated symptoms; however, some patients in this category can be managed by renal angio-infarction. A small subset of patients with solitary metastases may benefit from nephrectomy and resection of the metastatic lesion, based on a reported survival rate of up to 30–35%.

ADJUVANT SURGERY AND IMMUNOTHERAPY

There is currently an increasing interest in the use of adjunctive nephrectomy in combination with promising new immunotherapeutic regimes in an attempt to prolong longevity in patients with metastatic renal cell carcinoma. In this setting, adjuvant nephrectomy is being evaluated as a strategy for improving response rates by reducing overall tumor burden and, in some cases, by providing immunore-

active cells for therapy. Immune responses are often deficient in cancer patients, as shown by a delayed-type hypersensitivity reaction, decreased lymphocyte cytolytic function and a decreased lymphocyte proliferation response. Modern immunotherapy aims to bolster immune responses to the tumor (Figure 59). Another role for adjuvant surgery is in patients with residual or recurrent metastatic renal cell carcinoma after an initial response to nephrectomy and immunotherapy. Recent reports suggest that survival can be prolonged by surgical excision of such residual metastatic lesions in selected patients. Kim and colleagues have reported 11 patients with a partial response to nephrectomy and interleukin-2-based therapy; all of these individuals were alive and disease-free after a median follow-up of 21 months. Others have reported similarly encouraging results. It seems likely that surgery will be increasingly performed as an adjunct to either immunotherapy or gene therapy (Figure 60), but randomized, controlled studies will be needed to clarify the most useful integration of these treatment measures.

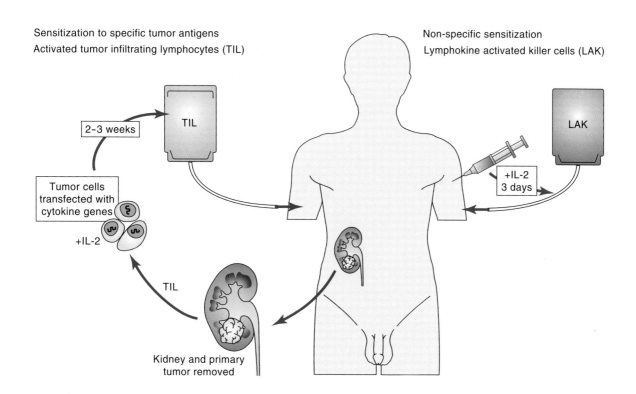

Figure 59 Immunotherapy for renal cell carcinoma: transfected tumor cells provoke an immune response against residual cancer cells

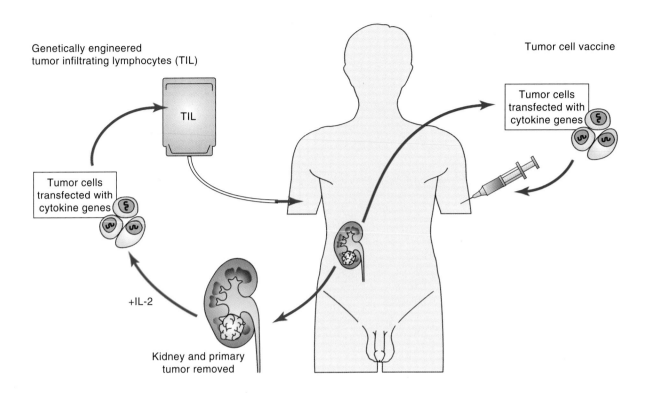

Figure 60 Gene therapy for renal cell carcinoma

FURTHER READING

Angermeier KW, Novick AC, Streem SB, Montie JE. Nephron-sparing surgery for renal cell carcinoma with venous involvement. *J Urol* 1990;144:1352–5

Broder S, Waldmann TA. Medical progress: The suppressor-cell network in cancer. *N Engl J Med* 1978;299:1281–4

Butler B, Novick AC, Miller D, Campbell SC, Licht MR. Management of small unilateral renal cell carcinomas: radical versus nephron-sparing surgery. *Urology* 1995;45:34–40; Discussion 40–1

Campbell SC, Novick AC, Streem SB, Klein EA. Management of renal cell carcinoma with coexistent renal artery disease. *J Urol* 1993;150:808–13

Campbell SC, Novick AC, Streem SB, Klein E, Licht M. Complications of nephron-sparing surgery for renal tumors. *J Urol* 1994;151:1177–80

Cheng WS, Farrow GK, Zincke H. The incidence of multicentricity in renal cell carcinoma. *J Urol* 1991;146:1221–3

Eggermont AM, Steller EP, Sugarbaker PH. Laparotomy enhances intraperitoneal tumor growth and abrogates the effects of interleukin-2 and lymphokine-activated killer cells. *Surgery* 1987;102:71–8

Fleischmann JD, Kim B. Interleukin-2 immunotherapy followed by resection of residual renal cell carcinoma. *J Urol* 1991;145:938–41

Fowler JE Jr. Nephrectomy in metastatic renal cell carcinoma. *Urol Clin North Am* 1987;14:749–56

Goldfarb DA, Novick AC, Lorig R, *et al*. Magnetic resonance imaging for assessment of vena caval tumor thrombi: a comparative study with vena cavography and CT scanning. *J Urol* 1990:144:1100–3

Guiliani I, Giberti C, Martorama G, *et al*. Radical extensive surgery for renal cell carcinoma: long-term results and prognostic factors. *J Urol* 1990;143:468–73

Kim B, Louis AC. Surgical resection following interleukin-2 therapy for metastatic renal cell carcinoma prolongs remission. *Arch Surg* 1992;127:1343–9

Konnack JW, Grossman HB. Renal cell carcinoma as an incidental finding. *J Urol* 1985;134:1094–6

Libertino JA, Zinman L, Watkins E. Long-term results of resection of renal cell cancer with extension into inferior vena cava. *J Urol* 1987;137:21–4

Licht MR, Novick AC. Nephron-sparing surgery for renal cell carcinoma. *J Urol* 1993;149:17

Licht MR, Novick AC, Goormastic M. Nephron-sparing surgery in incidental versus suspected renal cell carcinoma. *J Urol* 1994;152:39–42

Long JP, McClellan MW, Alexander RB, *et al*. The management of isolated renal recurrence of renal cell carcinoma following complete response to interleukin-2-based immunotherapy. *J Urol* 1993;150:176–8

Marcus SG, Choyke PL, Reiter R, et al. Regression of metastatic renal cell carcinoma after cytoreductive nephrectomy. J Urol 1993;150:463–6

Mitzoguchi H, O'Shea JJ, Longo DL, et al. Alterations in signal transduction molecules in T-lymphocytes from tumor-bearing mice. Science 1992;253:1795–8

Morgan WR, Zincke H. Progression and survival after renal-conserving surgery for renal cell carcinoma: experience in 104 patients and extended follow-up. J Urol 1990;144:852–7; Discussion 857–8

Mukamel E, Konichezky K, Engelstein D, Servadio C. Incidental small renal tumors accompanying clinically overt renal cell carcinoma. J Urol 1988;140:22–4

Naito S, Kimiya K, Sakarnoto N, et al. Prognostic factors and value of adjunctive nephrectomy in patients with stage IV renal cell carcinoma. Urology 1991;37:95–9

Neves RJ, Zincke H. Surgical treatment of renal cancer with vena cava extension. Br J Urol 1987;59:390–5

Nissenkorn I, Bernheim J. Multicentricity in renal cell carcinoma. J Urol 1995;153:620–2

Novick AC, Kaye M, Cosgrove DM, et al. Experience with cardiopulmonary bypass and deep hypothermic circulatory arrest in the management of retroperitoneal tumors with large vena caval thrombi. Ann Surg 1990;212:472–6

Novick AC, Streem SB. Long-term follow-up after nephron-sparing surgery for RCC in VHL disease. J Urol 1992;147:1488

Novick AC, Gephardt G, Guz B, Steinmuller D, Tubbs RR. Long-term follow-up after partial removal of a solitary kidney. N Engl J Med 1991;35:105–62

Novick AC. Partial nephrectomy for renal cell carcinoma. Urology 1995;46:149–52

O'Dea MJ, Zincke H, Utz DC, et al. The treatment of renal cell carcinoma with solitary metastasis. J Urol 1978; 120:540–2

Rackley R, Novick AC, Klein E, et al. The impact of adjuvant nephrectomy on multimodality treatment of metastatic renal cell carcinoma. J Urol 1994;152:1399–403

Robey EL, Schelhammer PF. The adrenal gland and renal cell carcinoma: is ipsilateral adrenalectomy a necessary component of radical nephrectomy? J Urol 1986; 135:453–5

Robson CJ, Churchill BM, Anderson W. The results of radical nephrectomy for renal cell carcinoma. J Urol 1969;101:297–303

Sella A, Swanson DA, Ro JY, et al. Surgery following response to interferon-a-based therapy for residual renal cell carcinoma. J Urol 1993;149:19–21

Siminovitch JP, Montie J, Straffon RA. Lymphadenectomy in renal adenocarcinoma. J Urol 1982;27:1090–1

Skinner DB, Colvin RB, Vermillion DC, et al. Diagnosis and management of renal carcinoma: a clinical and pathologic study of 309 cases. Cancer 1971;28:1165–77

Skinner DG, Pritchett TR, Lieskovsky G, et al. Vena caval involvement by renal cell carcinoma. Surgical resection provides meaningful long-term survival. Ann Surg 1989;210:387–92

Smith SI, Bosniak MA, Megibow AJ, Hulnick DR, Horii SC, Raghavendra BN. Renal cell carcinoma: earlier discovery and increased detection. Radiology 1989;170:699–703

Spencer WF, Linehan WM, Walther MM, et al. Immunotherapy with interleukin-2 and a-interferon in patients with metastatic renal cell cancer with in situ primary cancers: a pilot study. J Urol 1992;117:24–30

Steinbach F, Stockle M, Muller SC, et al. Conservative surgery of renal cell tumors in 140 patients: 21 years of experience. J Urol 1992;148:24–9; Discussion 29–30

Steinbach F, Novick AC, Shoskes D. Renal transplantation in patients with renal cell carcinoma and von Hippel Lindau disease. Urology 1994;44:760–3

Steinbach F, Novick AC, Zincke H, et al. Treatment of renal cell carcinoma in von Hippel Iindau disease: a multicenter study. J Urol 1995;153:1812–16

Thompson IM, Peck M. Improvement in survival of patients with renal cell carcinoma: the role of the serendipitously detected tumor. J Urol 1988;140:487–90

Tolia BM, Whitmore WF Jr. Solitary metastasis from renal cell carcinoma. J Urol 1975;114:836–8

Trindade JC, Rangel MC, Ross JR, et al. Influence of nephrectomy on the growth of a murine Wilms tumor. A study using parabiotic rats. J Urol 1990;144:418–21

von Eschenbach AC, Avallone A, Price J, et al. The biology of renal cancer: the influence of nephrectomy. Eur Urol 1990;18(Suppl 2):40–1

Walther MM, Alexander RB, Weiss GH, et al. Cytoreductive surgery prior to interleukin-2-based therapy in patients with metastatic renal cell carcinoma. Urology 1993;42:250–8

4

Bladder cancer

Transitional cell carcinoma is by far the most frequently encountered form of bladder cancer. Although most cases are sporadic, the disease is strongly associated with smoking as well as with certain occupations, including the aniline dye and rubber industries. In endemic areas, such as Egypt and around Lake Victoria, chronic schistosomal infections are associated with an increased risk of squamous cell carcinoma of the bladder.

DIAGNOSIS AND STAGING

The majority of bladder cancers present with painless hematuria; a smaller proportion have irritative voiding symptoms and dysuria, which may some-times be misinterpreted as bladder outflow obstruction. More work is required to educate the public about the significance of the painless passage of blood in the urine in order to facilitate earlier diagnosis and treatment of bladder cancer.

The investigations of choice are an intravenous urogram (IVU) followed by cystoscopy. In patients with irritative voiding and dysuria, a urine cytology can be helpful in distinguishing carcinoma *in situ* from the much more common condition of benign prostatic hyperplasia with bladder outflow obstruction and/or urinary tract infection. A urine culture will exclude the latter and may confirm microscopic hematuria. The IVU may reveal a space-occupying lesion in the bladder (Figure 61), and is more

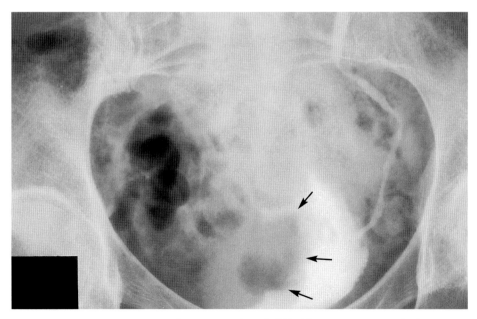

Figure 61 Intravenous urogram showing a right-sided bladder tumor (arrowed) obstructing the right ureter

sensitive than ultrasound in detecting associated transitional cell lesions in the renal pelvis or ureters.

Cystoscopy provides the definitive diagnosis and permits histological evaluation of the resected tissue. Of all investigations, this provides the most helpful information concerning future management. In this respect, both histological grade and stage are extremely important, especially the presence or absence of muscle invasion. A diagram illustrating the staging of transitional cell carcinoma may be found in Figure 62.

Grade 1 pTa tumors are generally not dangerous and are low risk for progression. Grade 2 pT1b tumors have a relatively low risk but should still be considered to have a potentially sinister prognosis. Grade 3 tumors, or any cancers which exhibit evidence of muscle invasion in pathological sections, should be considered potentially lethal and managed accordingly (Figure 63). Any associated carcinoma

in situ should be carefully noted since it may influence both the prognosis and the modality of treatment deployed (Figure 64).

After resection, staging investigations may include a CT scan to assess the depth and extent of muscle invasion and to identify any possible lymph node metastases (Figure 65). MRI scanning may achieve higher-resolution images, but has not been found to be greatly superior in clinical practice.

TREATMENT OPTIONS

The treatment options for patients with transitional cell carcinoma are illustrated in two decision diagrams (Figures 66 and 67). Many patients (> 80%) with transitional cell carcinoma can be managed simply by initial transurethral resection (Figure 68) and cystoscopic surveillance. In those

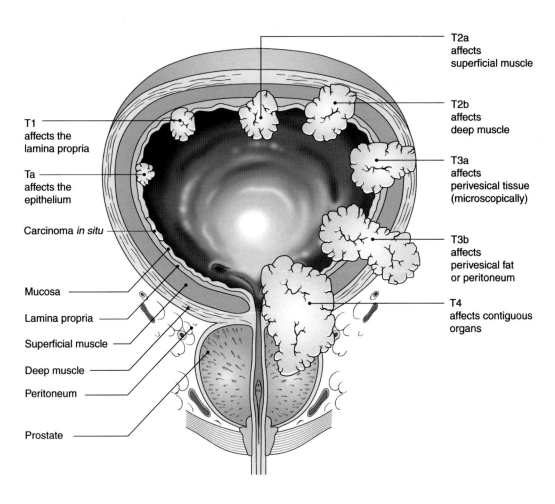

a

Figure 62 (a) Staging diagram of transitional cell carcinoma

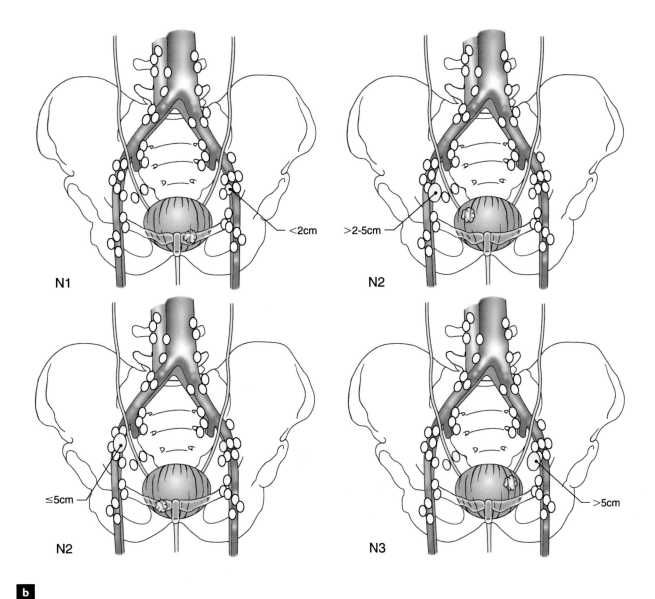

N1

<2cm

N2

>2-5cm

N2

≤5cm

N3

>5cm

Figure 62 (b) Diagram to illustrate how lymph node metastases from transitional cell carcinoma are staged

patients with G1 pTa lesions which are clear at 3 months, the cystoscopic interval can be increased quite rapidly. By contrast, those with single or multiple recurrences at 3 months are at significantly higher risk of disease progression. If there is doubt about the depth or presence of muscle invasion, rebiopsy of the tumor base may sometimes be required. Intravesical chemotherapy, with, for example, mitomycin C, has been shown to decrease the recurrence rate, but does not decrease progression or improve survival. Intravesical bacillus Calmette–Guérin (BCG) (six treatments over 6 weeks), however, does appear to decrease recurrence rate and can improve survival, especially in patients with carcinoma *in situ* present on biopsies adjacent to the tumor itself. Maintenance BCG can be given as three further treatments over 3 weeks after 6 months and has been shown to prolong the response. However, BCG treatment does carry a significant toxicity, and most patients experience frequency and dysuria for some weeks during and after therapy. Since live attenuated organisms are used, systemic BCG infections are a risk, and therapy after biopsy or resection should always be delayed until adequate mucosal healing has occurred to minimize this risk. Cystoscopic surveillance should usually be

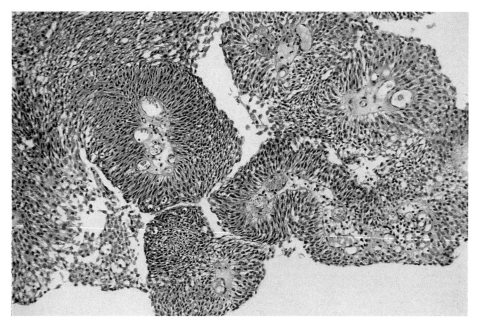

Figure 63 (a) Histology of grade 1 (well-differentiated) transitional cell carcinoma

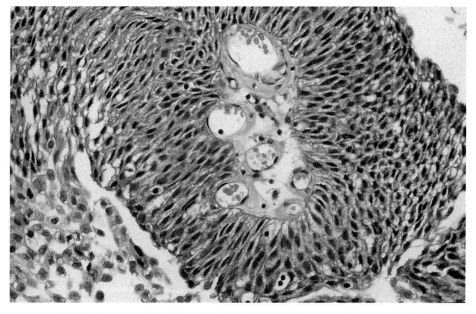

Figure 63 (b) Higher-power histology of grade 1 (well-differentiated) transitional cell carcinoma

continued until the patient has been clear of recurrences for at least 5 years or even longer.

EXTERNAL BEAM RADIOTHERAPY

External beam radiotherapy is a valuable treatment option for patients with muscle invasive bladder cancer, especially those older patients with significant co-morbidity in whom surgery is high risk. A total of 7000 cGy are usually administered in fractional doses (Figure 69). Toxicity includes urinary frequency, hematuria and dysuria, as well as proctitis with rectal bleeding. Response rates are in the order

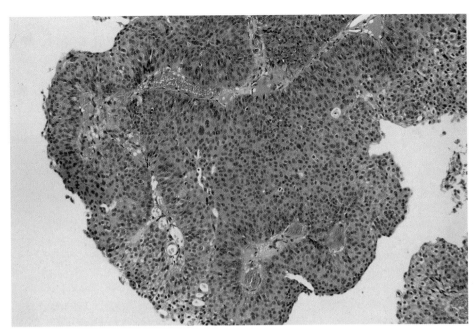

Figure 63 (c) Histology of grade 2 (moderately well-differentiated) transitional cell carcinoma

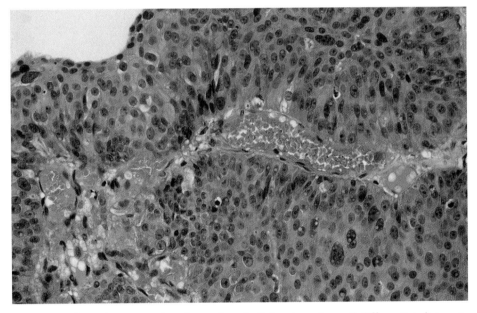

Figure 63 (d) Higher-power histology of grade 2 (moderately, well-differentiated) transitional cell carcinoma

of 50–70%, depending on the size and the aggressiveness and stage of the tumor.

Cystectomy

The indications for cystectomy include:

- Muscle invasive cancer

- Multiple recurrent superficial transitional cell carcinoma

- Superficial cancer with aggressive histology (e.g. lymphatic or perivascular invasion)

- Carcinoma *in situ* resistant to BCG

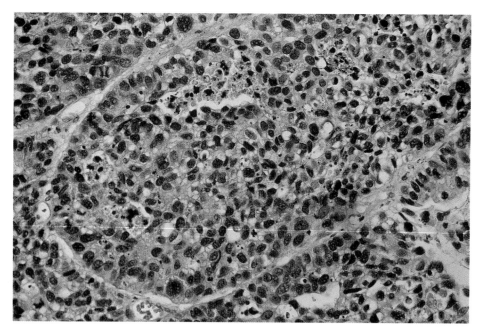

Figure 63 (e) Histology of grade 3 (poorly differentiated) transitional cell carcinoma

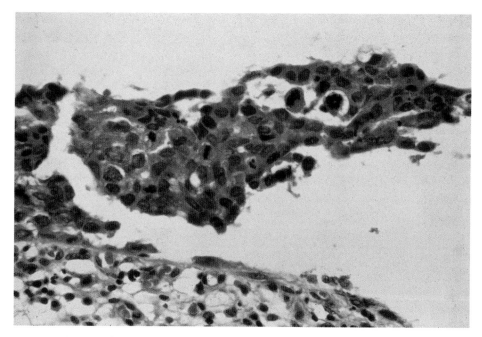

Figure 64 Histopathology of carcinoma *in situ* of the bladder

- Carcinoma *in situ* penetrating deep into prostatic ducts

- High-grade transitional cell carcinoma not accessible to adequate transurethral resection of bladder tumor

The procedure is performed through a lower midline abdominal incision. Bilateral obturator lymph node sampling is performed and the ureters are identified and encircled with slings, at the level of the pelvic brim, before being divided. The anterior dissection is taken down to the prostato–urethral junction, which may be dealt with in the same manner as a radical prostatectomy (Figure 70). The dorsal venous complex is secured and the urethra divided. The rectourethralis muscles are divided to open up the plane between the prostate and the

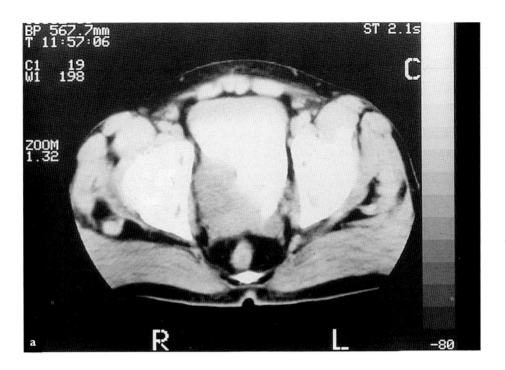

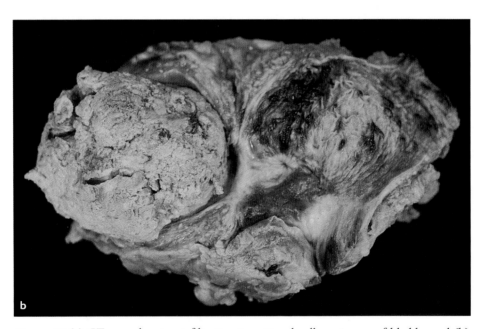

Figure 65 (a) CT scan showing infiltrating transitional cell carcinoma of bladder and (b) pathological specimen showing transitional cell tumor in a diverticulum

rectum. Attention is then paid to the posterior dissection. The peritoneum is divided at the junction between the bladder and the rectum and the space between these two structures developed. The lateral pedicles containing the superior and inferior vesical vessels are secured and divided, and the cysto-prostatectomy specimen sent for histological examination (Figure 65).

An ileal loop is the most tried and tested method of urinary diversion (Figure 71). A loop of ileum is isolated and bowel continuity restored. An anastomosis is then created between the ureters and the proximal end of the ileal loop, using 6 or 8F silicone tubing as stents. The distal end of the loop is brought out through the abdominal wall, usually in the right

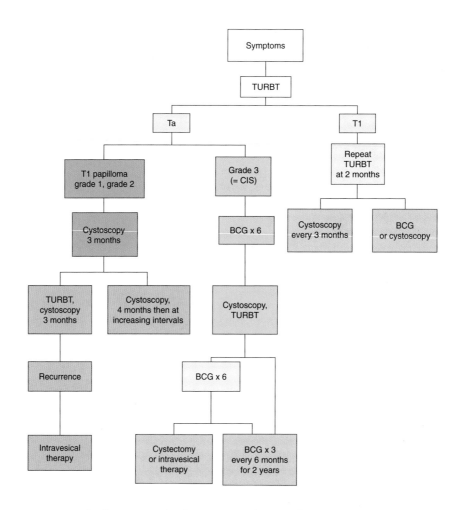

Figure 66 Superficial transitional cell carcinoma: decision diagram. TURBT, transurethral resection of bladder tumor; CIS, carcinoma *in situ*; BCG, bacillus Calmette–Guerin

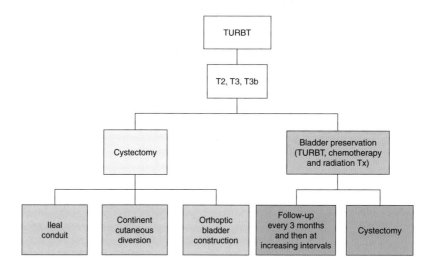

Figure 67 Muscle invasive bladder cancer: desicion diagram. TURBT, transurethral resection of bladder tumor

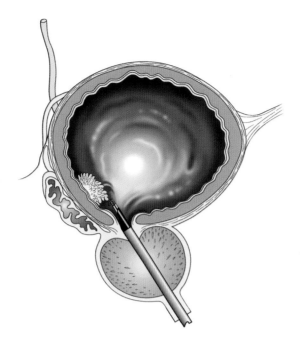

Figure 68 Transurethral resection of bladder tumor (TURBT)

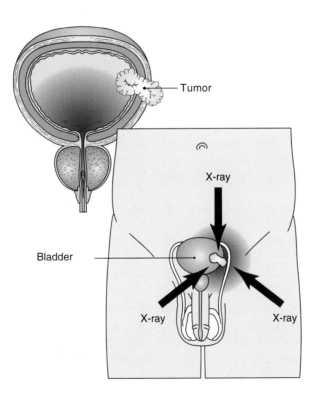

Figure 69 External beam radiotherapy: conformal planning allows maximum dosage to the tumor

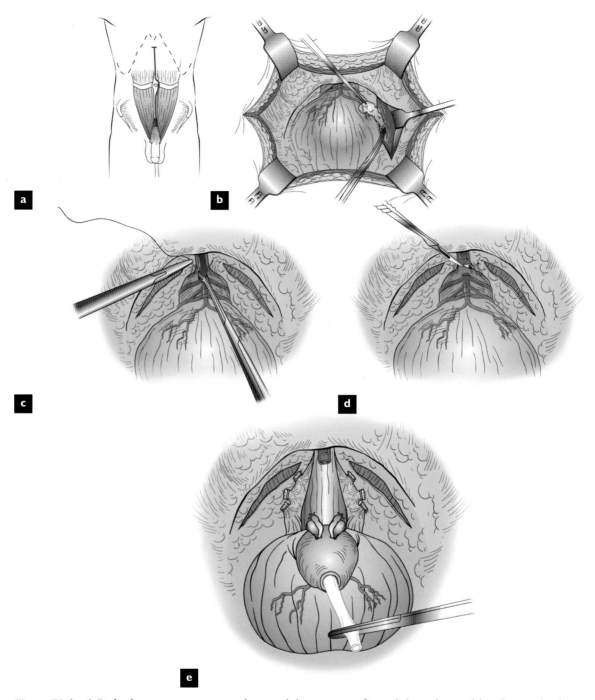

Figure 70 (a–e) Radical cystoprostatectomy: the apical dissection performed through a mid-line longitudinal incision

iliac fossa. A pelvic wound drain is placed and the wound closed in layers.

An alternative to the ileal loop, which, of course, requires the patient to wear a bag constantly, is a continent cutaneous diversion. The most experience has been gained with the Koch pouch, which uses an inverted ileal segment as a catheterizable nipple valve (Figure 72). Although these can function satis-

factorily, there is a significant revision rate because of either loss of continence of the valve or difficulty in achieving catheterization.

If the patient is very averse to the necessity for a urine-collecting bag, then a continent neobladder is sometimes the best option, provided that there is no distal disease extension down the urethra. A cysto-prostatectomy is performed, as described above, with

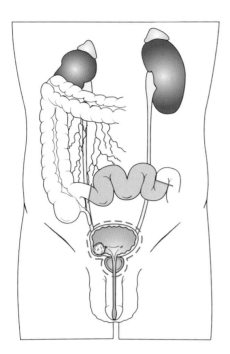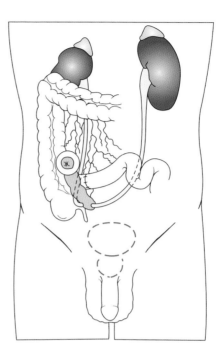

Figure 71 Ileal loop diversion: a small bowel segment is isolated and the continuity of the ileum restored. The ureters are then implanted into the proximal end of the ileal loop

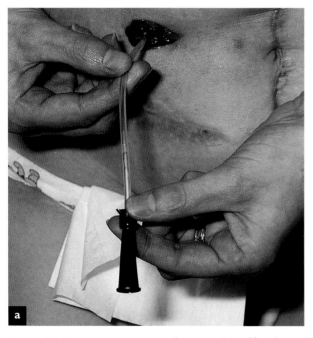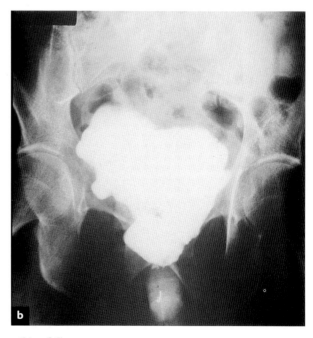

Figure 72 Cutaneous continent diversion (a) self-catheterization; (b) a follow-up cystogram

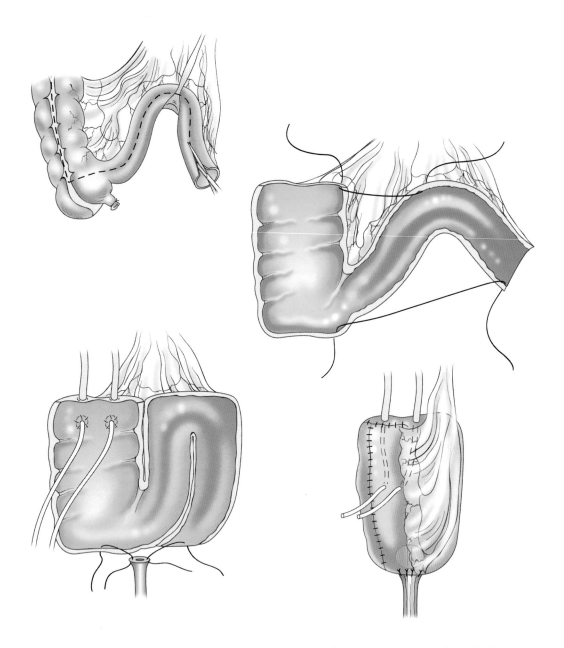

Figure 73 Neobladder formation using ileum, showing reimplantation of intubated ureters and urethral anastomosis

careful preservation of the urethra. A longer segment of bowel is then isolated and bowel continuity restored. A pouch is then created and ureters implanted over 8F stents. The urethra is then anastomosed to the neobladder over a 20F urethral catheter (Figure 73). A suprapubic catheter is also placed, together with an abdominal drain.

Results from this procedure are usually good, although there is a significant risk of distant recurrence of cancer. Urinary continence by day is usually excellent, but nocturnal eneuresis may be persistent and troublesome.

Treatment of transitional cell carcinoma involving the upper urinary tract

Transitional cell carcinoma can involve the ureter and/or the renal pelvis of either kidney. The diagnosis may be apparent on an IVU, but retrograde ureterography or ureteroscopy may be necessary to confirm the diagnosis. Treatment is usually by

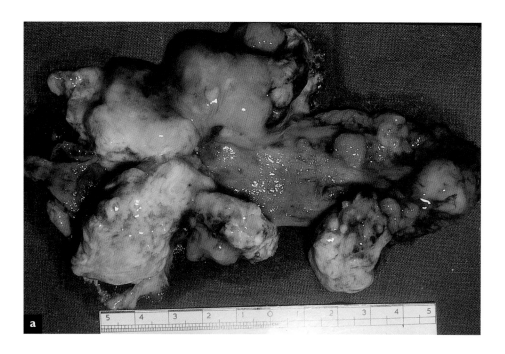

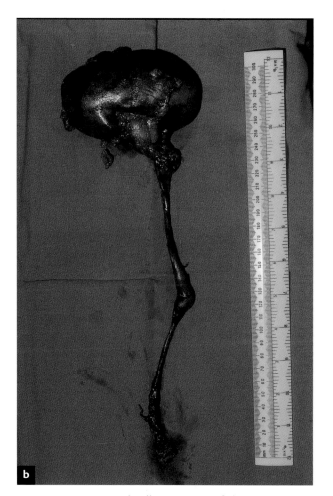

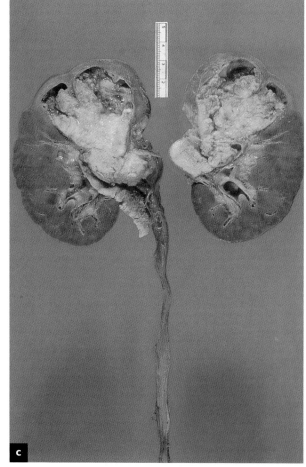

Figure 74 Transitional cell carcinoma of the upper urinary tract. (a) and (b) pathological specimens illustrating ureteric tumors; (c) transitional cell carcinoma in upper pole of kidney

nephroureterectomy, provided that the opposite kidney and ureter are unaffected (Figure 74) .

Treatment of metastatic disease

Metastatic bladder cancer is a difficult disease to eradicate. Deposits may occur in lungs, lymph nodes, other soft tissues or bones. Responses to chemotherapy may occur, but these are usually temporary and cure is seldom achieved. Palliative radiotherapy may be helpful if painful bone metastases are present.

FURTHER READING

Ali-EI-Dein, EI-Sobky E, Hohenfellner M, Ghoneim MA. Orthotopic bladder substitution in women: functional evaluation. *J Urol* 1999;161:1875–80

Cheng L, Weaver AM, Neumann AM, Scherer BG, Bostwick DG. Substaging of T1 bladder carcinoma based on the depth of invasion as measured by micrometer. *Cancer* 1999;86:1035–43

Cheng L, Bostwick OO. Progression of T1 bladder tumors: better staging or better biology? *Cancer* 1999;86:910–12

Epstein JI, Amin MB, Reuter VR, Mostofi FK, Bladder Consensus Conference Committee. The World Health Organization/International Society of Urological Pathology consensus classification of urothelial (transitional cell) neoplasms of the urinary bladder. *Am J Surg Pathol* 1998;22:1435–48

Freeman JA. Esrig D, Stein JP, *et al*. Radical cystectomy for high-risk patients with superficial bladder cancer in the era of orthotopic urinary reconstruction. *Cancer* 1995;76:833–9

Hautmann RE, De Petriooni A, Gottfried HW, Kleinschmidt K, Mattes AT, Paiss T. The ileal neobladder: complications and functional results in 363 patients after 11 years of followup. *J Urol* 1999;161:422–8

Herr HW. Extravesical tumor relapse in patients with superficial bladder tumors. *J Clin Oncol* 1998;16:1099–102

Herr HW, Bajorin OF, Scher HI. Neoadjuvant chemotherapy and bladder-sparing surgery for invasive bladder cancer: ten-year outcome. *J Clin Oncol* 1998;16:1298–301

Herr HW. The value of a second transurethral resection in evaluating patients with bladder tumor. *J Urol* 1999;162:74–6

Herr HW, Relrter YE. Progression of T1 bladder tumors: better staging or better biology? *Cancer* 1999;86:908–9

Kilbridge KL, Kantoff P. Intravesical therapy for superficial bladder cancer: is it a wash? *J Clin Oncol* 1994;12:1–4

Koch MO, Smith JA Jr. Influence of patient age and comorbidity on outcome of a collaborative care pathway after radical prostatectomy and cystoprostatectomy. *J Urol* 1996;155:1681–4

Lamm DL, Blumenstein BA, Crawford ED, *et al*. Randomized intergroup comparison of bacillus Calmette-Guerin immunotherapy and mitomycin C chemotherapy prophylaxis in superficial transitional cell carcinoma of the bladder. *Urol Oncol* 1995;1:119–26

Martins FE, Bennett CJ, Skinner D. Options in replacement cystoplasty following radical cystectomy: high hopes for successful reality. *J Urol* 1995;153:1363–72

McCaffrey JA, Bajorin OF, Scher HI, Bosi GJ. Combined modality therapy for bladder cancer. *Oncology* 1997;11:18–26

Pawinski A, Sylvester R, Kurth KH, *et al*. A combined analysis of European Organization for Research and Treatment of Cancer, and Medical Research Council randomized clinical trials for the prophylactic treatment of stage TaT1 bladder cancer. *J Urol* 1996;156:1934–41

Saxman SB, Propert KJ, Einhom LH, *et al*. Long-term follow-up of a phase III intergroup study of cisplatin alone or in combination with methotrexate, vinblastine, and doxorubicin in patients with metastatic urothelial carcinoma: a cooperative group study. *J Clin Oncol* 1997;15:2564–9

Tolley DA, Parmar MKB, Grigof KM, *et al*. The effect of intravesical mitomycin C on recurrence of newly diagnosed superficial bladder cancer: a further report with 7 years of follow-up. *J Urol* 1996:155:1233–8

5

Testicular cancer

EPIDEMIOLOGY

Testicular cancer usually affects younger men. Since the mid-twentieth century the incidence has been rising progressively for reasons that are still unclear. A history of an undescended testis, or of maternal treatment with progestogens during pregnancy, constitute the main risk factors.

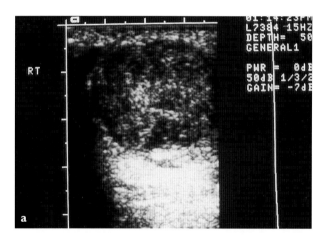

DIAGNOSIS

Testicular tumors usually present as painless, solid intratesticular masses. Much less commonly, they present as metastatic lesions in the paraaortic nodes or chest and the primary is hard to locate. For the purpose of treatment, the major histological classification is either seminoma or mixed germ cell tumor (teratoma).

Pre-operative tests should include a chest X-ray and serum tumor markers, β-human chorionic gonadotropin (β-hCG) and α-fetoprotein. Ultrasound of the testis usually confirms a space-occupying lesion and helps to distinguish testicular cancer from epididymo-orchitis (Figure 75).

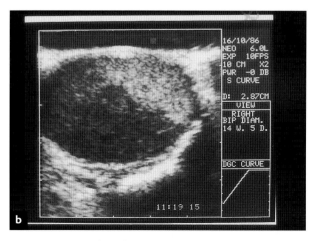

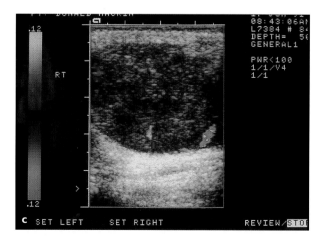

Figure 75 Testicular ultrasound showing testicular tumor: (a) teratoma, (b) seminoma, (c) Doppler ultrasound of teratoma

Staging investigations include an abdominal CT scan to detect involvement of paraaortic nodes. If these are positive, a chest CT may be helpful. Measurement of postoperative β-hCG and α-fetoprotein provides a means of identifying metastatic recurrence.

The clinical staging (Figure 76) is as follows:

- Stage 1: No metastases present

- Stage II: Clinically evident retroperitoneal metastases (Figure 77)

- Stage III: Distant metastases or lymph node involvement above the diaphragm (Figure 78)

TREATMENT OPTIONS

Orchiectomy

The testis with the malignancy present is removed through a groin incision. The cord should be clamped prior to mobilization to reduce the risk of cancer dissemination (Figure 79). In a minority of cases, a testicular prosthesis is used to replace the resected organ.

Treatment options differ significantly for seminoma and mixed germ cell tumors (Figure 80), because of the different chemo- and radiosensitivities of these tumor types.

Seminoma

- Clinical stage I: Retroperitoneal external beam radiotherapy to 2500–3000 cGy

- Clinical stage II: Systemic chemotherapy or (less effective) external beam radiotherapy

- Clinical stage III: Systemic chemotherapy

Mixed germ cell tumors

- Clinical stage I: Observation or retroperitoneal lymph node dissection (Figure 81)

- Clinical stage II: Either chemotherapy ± surgery for residual mass or retroperitoneal lymph node dissection and adjuvant chemotherapy

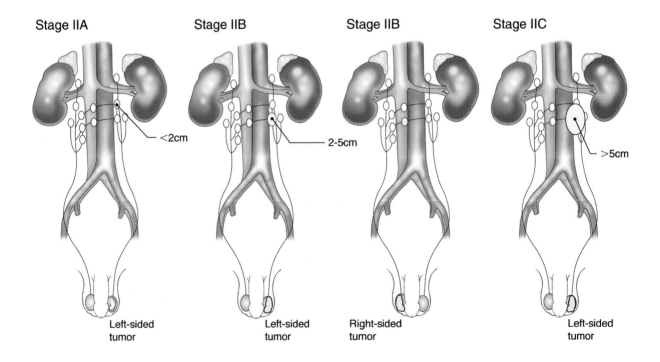

Figure 76 Staging diagram of testicular tumors

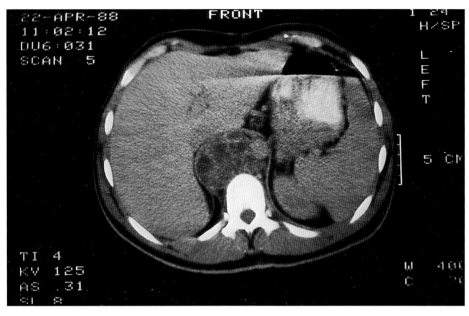

Figure 77 Cystic metastases from a testicular teratoma in retroperitoneum

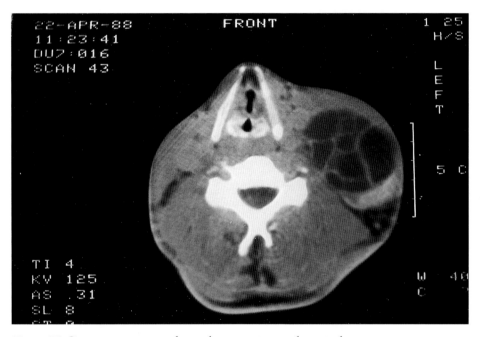

Figure 78 Cystic metastases in the neck in a patient with testicular teratoma

• Clinical stage III: Chemotherapy with resection of residual masses

Most recent studies favor surveillance and active treatment of recurrence over retroperitoneal lymph node dissection in mixed germ cell tumors. This is because of the morbidity associated with retroperitoneal lymph node dissection, even if a nerve-sparing technique is utilized, and the good outcomes achievable with surveillance alone. A decision diagram for the management of a solid intratesticular mass is illustrated in Figure 82.

Nowadays, the outcome from testicular cancer therapy is extremely good, with only the exceptional case failing to respond, giving resultant cure rates of more than 90%.

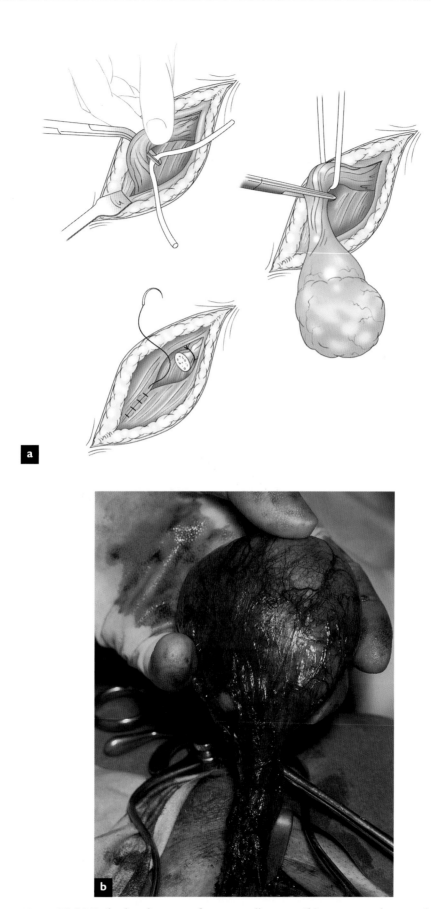

Figure 79 (a) Radical orchiectomy for germ cell cancer; (b) operative photograph

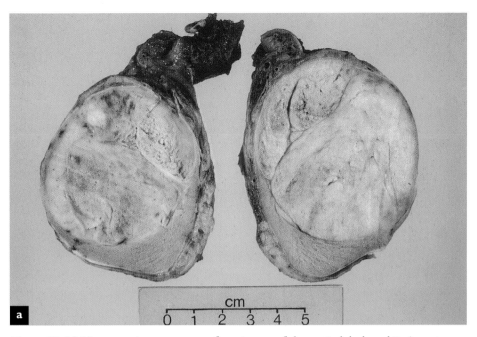

Figure 80 (a) Macroscopic appearance of seminoma of the testis: lobular white/gray tumor which may show foci of necrosis

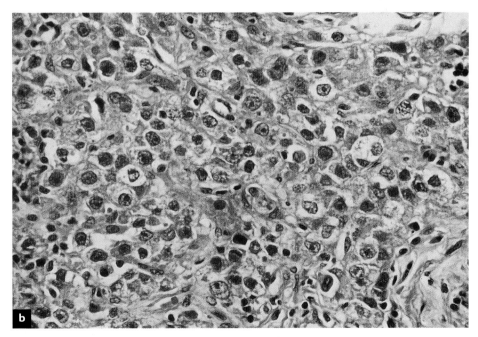

Figure 80 (b) Histology of seminoma of the testis: uniform infiltrate of polygonal cells with large nucleoli. Lymphocytes are commonly present   *Continued*

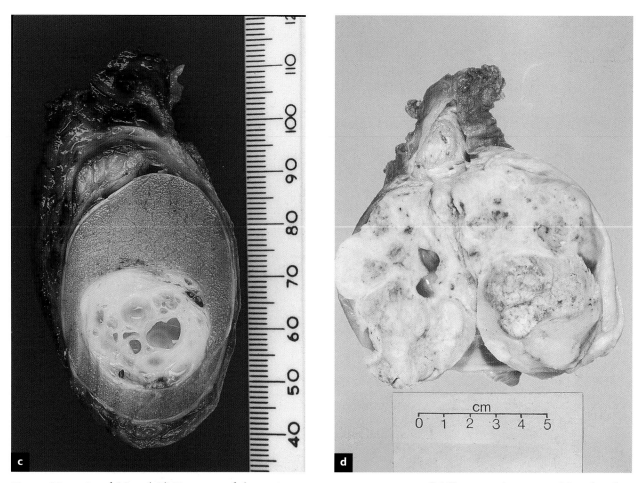

Figure 80 *continued* (c) and (d) Teratoma of the testis: macroscopic appearances of differentiated teratoma (c) and malignant teratoma intermediate (d) (WHO terminology, mixed germ cell tumor, teratoma and embryonal carcinoma)

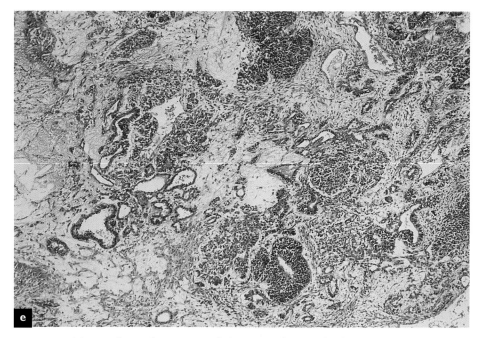

Figure 80 (e) Histology of teratoma of the testis showing both mature and immature components

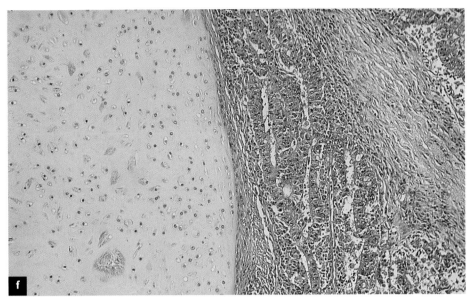

Figure 80 (f) Histology of a malignant teratoma intermediate of the testis showing cartilage formation on the left and undifferentiated teratoma (embryonal carcinoma) pattern on the right

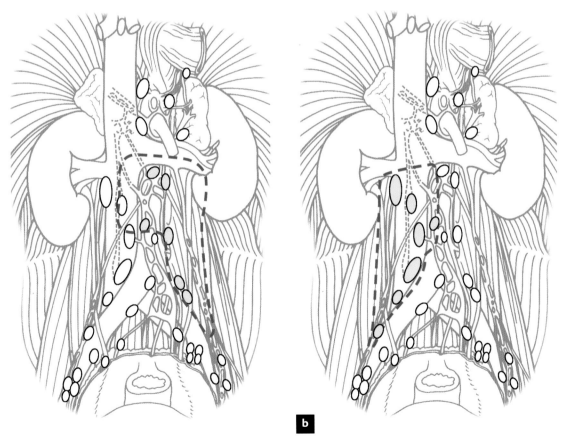

Figure 81 Retroperitoneal lymph node dissection: (a) left-sided tumor; (b) right-sided tumor

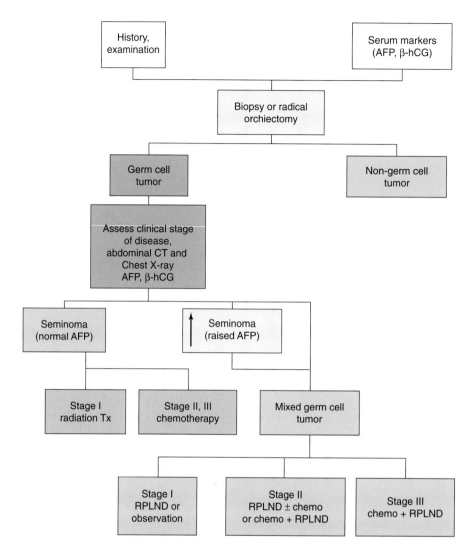

Figure 82 Decision diagram for the management of a solid testicular lesion. AFP, α-feto-protein; β-hCG, β-human chorionic gonadotropin; CT, computerized tomography; RPLND, retroperitoneal lymph node dissection; chemo, chemotherapy

FURTHER READING

Baniel J, Roth BJ, Foster AS, Donohue JP. Cost and risk benefit in the management of clinical stage II nonseminomatous testicular tumors. *Cancer* 1995;75:2897–903

Bosl GJ, Motzer RJ. Testicular germ-cell cancer. *N Engl J Med* 1997;331:242–53

Buohholz TA, Walden TL, Prestidge BR. Cost-effectiveness of post-treatment surveillance after radiation therapy for early stage seminoma. *Cancer* 1998;82:1126–33

Einhorn LH, Donohue JP. Advanced testicular cancer: update for urologists. *J Urol* 1998;160:1964–9

Hao D, Seidel J, Brant R, *et al.* Compliance of clinical stage I nonseminomatous germ cell tumor patients with surveillance. *J Urol* 1998;160:768–71

Heidenreich A, Sesterhenn IA, Mostofi FK, Moul JW. Prognostic risk factors that identify patients with clinical stage I nonseminomatous germ cell tumors at low risk and high risk for metastasis. *Cancer* 1998;83:1002–11

Herr HW, Sheinfeld J, Puc HS, *et al.* Surgery for a postchemotherapy residual mass in seminoma. *J Urol* 1997;157:860–2

International Germ Cell Cancer Collaborative Group. International germ cell consensus classification: a prognostic factor-based staging system for metastatic germ cell cancers. *J Clin Oncol* 1997;15:594–603

Warde P, Gospodarowicz M, Panzarella T, *et al.* Management of stage II seminoma. *J Clin Oncol* 1998;16:290–4

6

Penile cancer

Although penile cancer accounts for less than 1% of malignancies in western countries, the incidence is much higher in Asia, Africa and South America. Circumcision seems to be protective, and consequently neither Jews nor Muslims appear to be afflicted. Human papilloma virus (especially HDV-16) appears to be causative, while phimosis and poor penile hygiene are both associated with a higher prevalence.

More than 95% of penile cancers are squamous cell carcinomas (Figure 83). Pre-cancerous disorders include condylomata (especially Bushke–Lowenstein

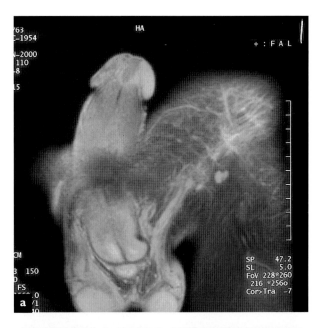

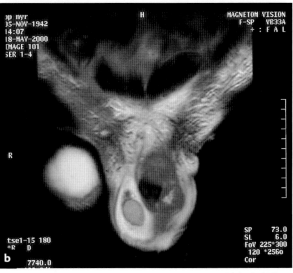

Figure 84 MRI of (a) penile squamous cell carcinoma involving glans, (b) involving corpus cavernosum

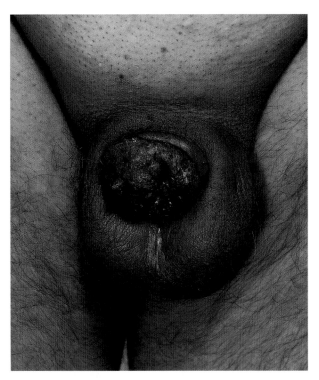

Figure 83 Macroscopic appearance of squamous cell carcinoma in the penis

giant condylomata). Carcinoma *in situ* (Bowen's disease/erythroplasia of Queryat) are also considered premalignant lesions.

Higher-grade tumors tend to metastasize to inguinal lymph nodes (initially superficial nodes, then deep inguinal and pelvic nodes). Nearly 50% of patients present with palpable nodes; however, nodal infection is extremely common and may often account for the swelling. Overall, pelvic lymph node dissection proves positive in around 20% of cases.

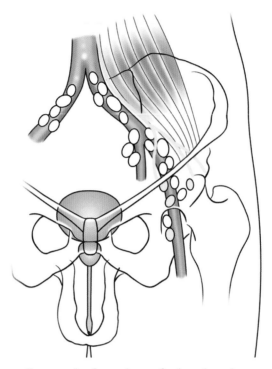

Figure 85 Diagram to illustrate the favored sites for lymph node metastases from penile squamous cell carcinoma

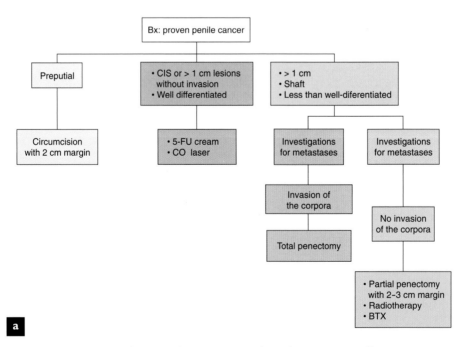

Figure 86 (a) Decision diagram of management of penile squamous cell carcinoma. CIS, carcinoma *in situ*; 5-FU, 5-fluorouracil; BTX, brachytherapy

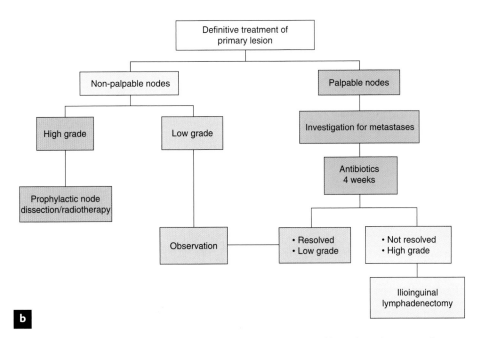

Figure 86 (b) Decision diagram of management of ileoinguinal lymph nodes in penile squamous cell carcinoma

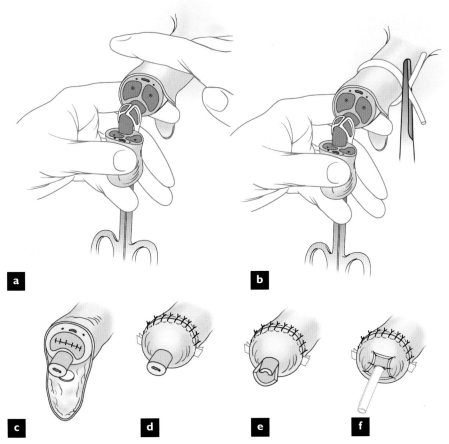

Figure 87 Penile amputation. (a) The corpora are divided and spongiosum preserved; (b) bleeding is reduced by a tourniquet; (c) a ventral skin flap is preserved; (d) the flap is brought dorsally, the urethra is delivered through the button-holed flap; (e) the urethra is spatulated; (f) a urethral catheter is retained

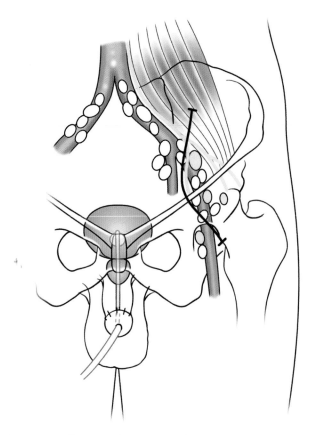

Figure 88 A diagram to illustrate the incision through which an inguinal lymph node dissection is performed

MRI (Figure 84) or ultrasound may sometimes facilitate local staging (Figure 85), but a biopsy of the lesion is required to confirm the diagnosis. A decision diagram for the management of penile squamous cell carcinoma is illustrated in Figure 86.

Treatment is usually by local excision with reconstruction of the penile urethra at the neomeatus (Figure 87). In cases where inguinal nodes are palpable, an inguinal lymphadenectomy may be required (Figure 88). Squamous cell cancers of the penis also respond to external beam radiotherapy or brachytherapy.

FURTHER READING

Chaudhary AJ, Ghosh S, Bhalavat RL, Kulkarni IN, Sequeira BV. Interstitial brachytherapy in carcinoma of the penis. *Strahlenther Onkol* 1999;175:17–20

Cubilla AL, Reuter VE, Gregoire L, *et al.* Basaloid squamous cell carcinoma: a distinctive human papilloma virus-related penile neoplasm: a report of 20 cases. *Am Surg Pathol* 1998;22:755–61

Davis JW, Schellhammer PF, Schlossberg SM. Conservative surgical therapy for penile and urethral carcinoma. *Urology* 1999;53:386–92

Derakshani PF, Neubauer S, Braun M, Bargmann H, Heidenreich A, Engelmann U. Results and 10-year follow-up in patients with squamous cell carcinoma of the penis. *Urol Int* 1999;62:238–44

Donnellan SM, Webb OR. Management of invasive penile cancer by synchronous penile lengthening and radical tumour excision to avoid perineal urethrostomy. *Aust NZ J Surg* 1998;68:369–70

Haas GP, Blumenstein BA, Gagliano RG, *et al.* Cisplatin, methotrexate and bleomycin for the treatment of carcinoma of the penis: a Southwest Oncology Group Study. *J Urol* 1999;161:1823–25

Han K, Brogle BN, Goydos J, Perrotti M, Cummings KB, Weiss RE. Lymphatic mapping and intraoperative lymphoscintigraphy for identifying the sentinel node in penile tumors. *Urology* 2000;55:582–5

Hoffman MA, Renshaw AA, *et al.* Squamous cell carcinoma of the penis and microscopic pathologic margins. *Cancer* 1999;85:1565–8

Horenblas S, Jansen L, Meinhardt W, Hoefnagel CA, de Jong D, Nieweg OE. Detection of occult metastasis in squamous cell carcinoma of the penis using a dynamic sentinel node procedure. *J Urol* 2000;163:100–4

Krieg R, Hoffman R. Current management of unusual genitourinary cancers. I. Penile cancer. *Oncology* 1999;13:1347–52

Kumar MPS, Ananthakrishnan N, Prema V. Predicting regional lymph node metastasis in carcinoma of the penis: a comparison between fine-needle aspiration cytology, sentinel lymph node biopsy and medial inguinal lymph node biopsy. *Br J Urol* 1998;81:453–7

Levi JE, Rahal P, Sarkis AS, *et al*. Human papillomavirus DNA and p53 status in penile carcinomas. *Int J Cancer* 1998;76:779–83

Micali G, Innocenzi D, Nasca MR, *et al*. Squamous cell carcinoma of the penis. *J Am Acad Derm* 1999;35:432–51

Shirahama T, Takemoto M, Nishiyama K, *et al*. A new treatment for penile conservation in penile carcinoma: a preliminary study of combined laser hyperthermia, radiation and chemotherapy. *Br J Urol* 1998;82:687–93

Skoog L, Collins BT, Tani E, *et al*. Fine needle aspiration cytology of penile tumors. *Acta Cytol* 1998;42:1336–40

Tietjen DN, Malek RS. Laser therapy of squamous cell dysplasia and carcinoma of the penis. *Urology* 1998;52:559–65

Concluding thoughts

Unfortunately, at the current incidence levels, one in three of us is destined eventually to suffer from some form of cancer. And since cancers of the urogenital tract are so common, the chances of it being a uro-oncological tumor are really rather high. The field of uro-oncology is wide and rapidly expanding. Accordingly, I have not attempted to illustrate every aspect in this slim book, but instead have focused on the more common oncological tumor types. I have also weighted the contents towards the more prevalent tumor sites. I hope the flavor that I have provided will stimulate the reader's appetite for further reading and more detailed study into these diseases that afflict so many people, but for which so much can be accomplished by timely diagnosis and skilful intervention.

Index